REWRITE
THE
MOTHER
CODE

From Sacrifice to Stardust –
A Cosmic Approach to Motherhood

BY DR. GERTRUDE LYONS

REWRITE THE MOTHER CODE

**RISE
BOOKS**

Jacket design and illustrations by Caitlin Keegan

Interior design by Laura Boyle

Library of Congress Cataloging-in-Publication Data

Available on request

ISBN 978-1-959524-12-0 (hardcover)

ISBN 978-1-959524-13-7 (e-book)

Printed in the United States of America

First Edition

10 9 8 7 6 5 4 3 2 1

Advance Praise for
Rewrite the Mother Code

"What a tremendous gift this book is to mothers, and to all humanity! *Rewrite the Mother Code* lays out how to shed the old, damaging stories of motherhood and actively step into mothering from our values, vision, and joy. This is a book to read before you become a mother, if you have young or grown children, or if you are in any role with kids. May this book become a companion and champion especially for all new mothers. It is a pathway for deep family, and global, healing."

—HeatherAsh Amara, author of *Warrior Goddess Training*
and *Wild, Willing, and Wise*

"*Rewrite the Mother* Code is an essential guide for any woman on a journey to and through mothering."

—Dr. Katie Bodendorfer Garner, Executive director of IAMAS
(International Association of Maternal Action and Scholarship)

"*Rewrite The Mother Code* speaks to the head and heart and helps awaken the nurturing abilities in all of us - including men. Gertrude has explored all aspects of the mothering journey and has brought to the surface many more ways for us to value all it takes conceive, create and give birth to our children. She emphasizes a return to the spiritual gifts of the natural birth process versus a less empowered reliance on modern medicine. You will understand and heal many aspects of your life reading this book and you will want to share many copies with your family and friends!"

—David Elliott, author of *Healing* and *The Reluctant Healer*

"This revelatory book was the guide I most needed as a young mother—and which I will be pressing into the hands of every expectant parent I know.

Gertrude Lyons gifts us life-changing wisdom as she helps us de-condition from our unconscious myths around mothering and give birth to a healing vision for ourselves, our children and the world. This is an essential, urgent book I hope everyone, everyone, reads and shares."

—Perdita Finn, author of *Way of the Rose, Take Back the Magic* and *Mothers of Magic*

"*Rewrite the Mother Code* is a catalyst for reimagining motherhood as a journey of transformation and self-discovery. Through powerful stories and timeless wisdom, it inspires readers to break free from limiting beliefs, trust their intuition, and embrace their full potential. This book is a profound invitation to redefine what it means to mother and create a new story for yourself and the world."

—Avanti Kumar-Singh, MD, Ayurveda Expert, Author of *The Longevity Formula* & *The Health Catalyst*, Host of The Healing Catalyst podcast

"Becoming a mother was one of the hardest things I ever did. I was completely unprepared for the eruption of the mother code in my psyche, telling me what kind of mother I had to be, nor was I ready for what the culture told me a good mother was—and wasn't. Dr. Lyons has written a profoundly important book to help you write a story of motherhood that serves *you* and your child so that you can have a whole-hearted whole-self motherhood. I wish I had this book all those years ago and I'm so happy my daughter will."

—Jennifer Louden, best-selling author of *The Woman's Comfort Book* and *Why Bother?*

"*Rewrite the Mother Code* by Dr. Gertrude Lyons is an essential, transformative guide that challenges and redefines our understanding of motherhood, humanity, and the act of nurturing. Lyons masterfully weaves poetry, guided meditation, history, storytelling, and reflective prose into a compelling journey of self-discovery. Through each page, readers are invited to explore the depths of their own psyche and awaken to new ways of thinking and being that are sorely needed in today's world. This book is not just a read; it's an immersive experience—one that calls for a shift in how we see ourselves and embrace the power of nurturing ourselves, others, all children and the world, moving far beyond traditional views of motherhood. Lyons' work feels timely, necessary, and nothing short of groundbreaking.

—Dr. Dominica McBride, founder and director of Become, author of *Becoming Change Makers: The Exquisite Path to Leadership and Liberation for Women of Color*

"A necessary and vital re-imagining of motherhood through Dr. Lyons radical and innovative theory and practice of *Rewriting the Mother Code.* The book opens up narrow conceptions of what mothering is to redefine and re-invent motherhood as site of empowerment for all who engage in mothering however it may be determined and experienced. The book rightly and per-suasively argues that this reimagining and rewriting must first and foremost begin with all of us, including mothers themselves, honouring, valuing, and supporting every mother. A splendidly insightful and hopeful book that envisions a more just and caring world for mothers and their families."

—Dr. Andrea O'Reilly, Founder of motherhood studies, maternal theory, and matricentric feminism and author of *In (M)otherwords: Writings on Mothering and Motherhood, 2009-2024* and *Matricentric Feminism: Theory, Activism, Practice*

"As a gay transgender father who has walked my own path of reimagining family, fertility, and selfhood, I was deeply moved by Dr. Gertrude Lyons' *Rewrite the Mother Code*…a must-read for anyone longing to connect with the sacred, healing power of mothering in all its forms."

—Trystan Reese, Author of *How We Do Family*

"Dr. Gertrude Lyons has written the book I wish I'd had at the start of my journey as a mother. Wise, worldly, and brimming with transformative teachings, it offers a wellspring of inspiration at the intersection of the mystical and the practical. Lyons guides us to connect with the divine wisdom within so we can transform life's hardships into healing and self-trust. More than a book, *Rewrite the Mother Code* is a revolutionary call to re-envision how we mother in all areas of our lives."

—Alexia Vernon, Speaking and Thought Leadership Expert, author of *Step into Your Moxie: Amplify Your Voice, Visibility, and Influence in the World*

"I wish I'd had this book to read when I was pregnant, in fact I wish I'd had it long before. And it isn't just for mothers. All of us have or had a mother, and live with the imprint not only of who and how she was but with how society sees motherhood in general. Reading the book really does rewrite a code, a code we weren't even conscious of having received but which definitely needed a modern — and a mystical — rewrite. Bravo to Gertrude Lyons for doing it. Many destinies will unfold differently because you did."

—Marianne Willamson, Marianne Williamson, New York Times bestselling author of *A Return to Love and A Woman's Worth*

"Dr. Gertrude Lyons has written a cosmic reclamation for the everywoman. *Rewrite the Mother Code* is more than a book about mothering. It's even more than a guide for women seeking deeper connection to their children and themselves. This book is a transcendent transmission, channeled from the author's personal motherhood journey as much as her deep spiritual wisdom, as she takes us on a profound inner voyage to heal, awaken and activate our collective feminine power at this time in humanity. As you read these pages, Dr. Lyons is here to help you remember—children or no children—that we are all on the same sisterhood team, and that within every woman exists every woman.

—Jessica Zweig, best-selling author of *The Light Work*, and *Be*.

To all the mothers and daughters in my mother line—whose wisdom is our legacy.

Contents

Introduction

Your first human home is a womb. You live inside another human's body. Cells multiply. Out of nowhere, in a dark, slippery, wet container, you become matter. You chose this human. You chose this womb.

You are spirit made manifest in the darkness. You hear the heartbeat. You become the sensations of your host. "Oh, this is what it is like to be human!" You are making yourself. She is making you. Everyone around you is forming you.

Light is masculine. Dark is feminine. Two forces that work together in harmony to bring forth life. The heat and warmth united within the darkness. No external light enters the sacred space of the womb. Only the spark of creation exists, putting form around the wisdom of the universe.

There are no mistakes, only learning. You know this as truth when you are in the womb, and then as you join humankind, it is yours to rekindle that flame repeatedly and ultimately connect back to the wisdom of your beginning.

Around the time my daughters reached high school, the fog began to lift. It was as if I stepped out of the land of the Faery Folk—the ancient and otherworldly place of enchantment. That parallel realm of motherhood was filled with allure and wonder, a place where time flowed differently and the rules of reality were altered. In legends, the land of the Faery folk is often described as a mystical journey where ordinary perceptions are heightened, and the boundaries between the physical and spiritual worlds blur. I found motherhood to feel much the same way.

The last thing I remembered before slipping into this parallel reality was that I was on a path of personal development, one which also included my husband and our newly growing family. It led us into unfamiliar internal territory—raw honesty, deep emotional expression, and spiritual exploration. It was risky stuff and out of the ordinary for the times.

We were making conscious, discerned choices around how we conceived and gave birth to our daughters. Our choices were making my family and friends uncomfortable, but they felt congruent with our values and my intuitive wisdom. When our daughters were babies, I was telling truths to my husband about how he was competing with me to be the better parent. I was uncovering painful wounds about beliefs I had that I'm not enough and could not nourish my infant sufficiently so she would thrive.

Then, in what felt like an instant (even though I know it happened over months and even years after our second daughter was born), the fog rolled in and got thicker and thicker. Now I was careful not to rock the boat with my husband. I started avoiding anything that sniffed of deeper inquiry into my past trauma and tried to maintain security in the messy disruptiveness of mothering. I was embarrassed to expose my crushing self-doubt and the not "enoughness" that motherhood brought up for me, so I started coasting. I didn't want to risk losing the financial security my husband was providing for me and our children.

I wanted things to be easy, safe, and comfortable—like in Faery Land. This identity as mother I thought would provide me with a sense of wholeness and purpose was kicking me in the ass. On the outside, I was doing all the right things, and I thought I was superior to the status quo. I was making self-aware and conscious choices. But my healing and transformation journey was fading to the background and I was losing myself in my children. My husband and I were parenting well together but after the first couple years it wasn't something that was bringing us closer or deepening our intimacy. It was a project, and that project was about the kids, not us. We were still doing couples coaching, but sessions were often conveniently focused on working through parenting issues.

As the fog thickened, my fresh, and hard-earned, belief in my value as a woman was getting less and less accessible. Instead of growing with my children, I was living through them and perpetuating an unhealthy cycle of instilling the belief that love and acceptance must be earned through performance. I grew up being the emotional caretaker of my parents and felt responsible for their happiness. And I was unknowingly putting that same burden onto my children.

The full truth of how far I had regressed into old patterns and behaviors did not reveal itself overnight. My first wake-up call was like a foghorn piercing the mist. It happened while my husband and I were participating in a yearly spiritual pilgrimage, a tradition we kept alive during our marriage.

You will hear about several such trips as my story unfolds on these pages. I am acutely aware that traveling the world as part of my spiritual seeking is a profound privilege. While I acknowledge gratitude for this privilege, I wasn't engaging in these trips as a vacation or for my benefit alone. I believed it was my responsibility to bring back and share the teachings, insights, blessings, and experiences I was granted—not as a travel log, but as a transmission that I hoped would inspire, guide, or help people meaningfully.

A collective energy aimed at healing, spiritual self-awareness, and personal transformation had ripple effects in and around the communities we were learning from.

It was in Katmandu, Nepal, that the pathway to my next level of growth was illuminated. With the Himalayan Mountains in the background, we met with several healers and visited sacred sites. Just what you might imagine in this place—fire healing, cosmic snake temple symbolizing the "All-in-All," the totality of existence, infinity, and the cyclic nature of the cosmos.

The pinnacle of this trip came when I was receiving a blessing from a Nepalese shaman who healed through her loving touch and hugs. It was profound. I melted in her arms and sobbed for what felt like an eternity but was probably only a few minutes. While I was held in the security of her embrace, I felt a calling. The invitation was to step out of my current, isolated comfort zone and into using my voice to speak from my head and heart as a critical thinker and intuitive healer. I was directed to do this first with myself then in my work and relationships.

Out of this, I did the unthinkable and said to everyone on the trip that I would engage in the study of motherhood as a vehicle for transformation and start the journey of earning my doctoral degree.

What the heck was I thinking? After nine years to complete two master's degrees, I had decided I was done with school! But this directive came from a transcended place inside of me, and while I almost pulled out several times before the quarter started, I ultimately decided to begin this new journey.

Over the next four years, I turned myself inside out and confronted false but ingrained beliefs around what I was capable of intellectually and creatively. In the process of "studying" the developmental opportunity in mothering, my defensive layers began to shed, and I came face-to-face with the truth that while I had started on the path of self-growth, I didn't commit to the process.

My doctoral journey transformed me, and I felt my dissertation was my third child. In this process, I birthed the Rewrite the Mother Code framework (although it would not be named for two more years). A few months before my doctoral defense, I was gifted with another mystical experience on the Mekong River in Laos. Our barge carried us to the Pak Ou Caves.

Originally an ancient temple space of the Khmu peoples dedicated to river spirits and nature deities, it has since become a resting place for broken Buddha statues—or as it was described to us, beautifully imperfect Buddha statues. There I was flooded, first with regret and remorse, and eventually with compassion for myself as a mother on her journey. As a force of four thousand statues strong, their collective energy created a sacred and healing place. Suddenly, I understood that the pain I experienced, the mistakes I made, and the regret I felt were beautiful, just as each individual statue was as or more beautiful broken than when it was whole.

The pain we experience as mothers is beautiful. It is an essential part of our journey. And while this pain is felt in unique ways by each woman, when bravely shared, it has the power to heal collectively. I hold we each carry a piece of universal pain and the expression of this pain has ripple effects, touching not only those closest to us but all of humanity.

Motherhood is a natural evolutionary and biological process, but not one I believe is intended to be carried out alone. In community with other women, we have space to learn and develop and fine-tune our innate capacity to love and care for our children and all children. Consider what it would be like if it was a commonly held tradition for the wise women in our Western culture to support women through the mothering process. What if children were raised by the community and not the isolated responsibility of one or two caregivers? What if all women were united as mothers and gave their full support to each other's mothering choices?

Welcome to Rewrite the Mother Code! A movement toward fulfilling these ideals can open the doors for women to take part in the abundance of the world and make sure everyone else experiences it. Mothers would feel valued and intrinsically aware that fostering their well-being is the keystone for conscious and harmonious living on Earth—a world where there are enough resources for everyone, all life is valued, and decisions are made with everyone's best interests in mind, not just a few.

You may be resonating with these ideas, or you may be saying to yourself, "Whoa! What the heck is happening! I thought this book was about how I could create a *personally* meaningful mothering experience. What's all this 'change the world' stuff?"

Well, it is about *all* of it! The personal and global go hand-in-hand, and I want you to know from the start that your personal journey matters in an even broader sense. Your desire to have a more nourishing, healing, and self-actualized experience in mothering is not only beneficial for you; the ripple effects and potential for a major shift in the collective consciousness around mothering is a bonus result of your efforts. By the simple fact that you have this book in your hands, you are already contributing to that shift inside and around you. It means you are anywhere from curious to adamant that things need to change—personally and/or collectively.

This book is not only for and about women mothering children, it is for and about all women and people who identify as women. As we will explore more deeply through these pages, I want to blur the lines that pigeonhole women into limited roles that ultimately disempower them. Rather than operating with a narrow conception of what mothering is, we will open ourselves up to what is possible when we realize that all women mother, and that mother energy is accessible to all of us—including men.

Speaking of men, I want to be clear that I am neither excluding them from the conversation nor diminishing their role. While I will address women predominantly, I not only want men to be included personally in ways that support them as fathers, but I also hope to provide an opening for them to use the creative power of mothering in their lives. In full transparency, I selfishly want to pull up the curtain and show what it takes for fathers to support and empower the women in their lives so they can embody the mothering experience.

I respect all personal pronouns and the choice to identify with the ones most resonant for each individual. For ease of reading, meaning no disrespect, I will mainly use she/her/hers. Similarly, my use of the terms masculine and feminine is not intended to denote gender, rather to represent qualities and values that coincide closely with the principles found in the Yin (feminine) Yang (masculine) symbol.

All people mother. We conceive. We create. We give birth to ideas, dreams, careers, children, and so much more. Whether you have kids or not, you are already a mother. You mother your career, your relationships, your dreams—and most importantly, you mother yourself.

In each chapter, I have included a ritual and a reflection. These are meant to give you space to pause and connect with yourself. After the introduction of the chapter, I offer a ritual or brief meditation that is loosely tied to the upcoming content, designed for you to drop in and experience the potency and clarity that rituals and meditations can bring to your day.

Then at the end of the chapter is a reflection to allow you to consider the material personally. These are suggestions, and there is no right or wrong way to engage with them. You always have full choice to play at whatever level you desire. And that desire may ebb and flow.

Sometimes, you may be drawn to do a deep dive with certain material or a particular ritual or reflection; other times, you may skip them entirely. And there may be times the book sits on your nightstand for days, weeks, and even months. Just having a book with inspirational content near you brings the energy into your space.

At the same time, I am an advocate for adding coaching and other supports to deepen your experience. Research shows that roughly 5-10% of readers experience change or transformation by reading alone. When you add a coaching and behavior-changing application, the impact increases to 30-50%. The most effective combination for transformational impact is education, practical application, and community support. Mostly I want you to have all the support you need to get the most out of this experience.

I suggest keeping a journal of your thoughts and feelings that emerge as you go through this book. Who knows what will get stirred for you. I hope a lot does! I hope these structures offer a safe space for you to liberate your mind and open your heart.

Let's dance around the fire and envision our dreams. Let's tell stories. Let's share wisdom. Let's impart knowledge. Let's light the inner spark of creation. Together, let us all—sisters, mothers, aunties, grandmother, daughters—gather by the fire and share stories of our births, of our lessons of mothering for everyone around us, including ourselves. Infants at our breasts. Children dance with the freedom only unburdened spirits know, untouched by the world's weight. Their movements flicker like wild flames—sacred, healing, and creative—until the overculture, as Clarissa Pinkola Estés describes, settles over them. This overculture, the dominant narrative of what is acceptable, teaches conformity over authenticity, dimming their brilliance. The vibrant flame fades, replaced by an artificial glow—a light that never shuts off, reflecting society's endless demands. Always on, but never warm, it offers no comfort—only expectation, leaving the soul restless, striving, and yet never truly fulfilled.

Dance with me in ceremony around the fire, casting off the overculture. We will alchemize together. Through the ring of fire, we will collectively birth a new revolution of empowered living, of embodied living. Solid in our form. Grounded in the earth. Sensitive to the air. Immersed in the water of our being. We come alive again. The blanket is removed, and we see the organic, natural light of the flame. Of our beating heart pulsing. Of our throat singing our own song.

Let's go to the river. Let's merge with the flow of the water. We are born out of the water and earth and the sun. Look at the resemblance! Look into the river, the fields, the desert, the mountains, the ocean, and see your reflection.

"Gosh you look so much like your Mother. The resemblance is uncanny!"

Let's jump in...

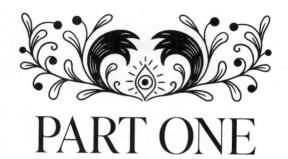

PART ONE

FIRST TRIMESTER

The Primordial Waters wash me to and fro.
Until I anchor and
fill the space
of your Eternity.
Where does Matter come from?
Building from within your being
I can't see you, but I know you.
We speak the language of the
Water
Air
Earth
Fire
Sky
Moon.
We know each other

from times past.
The waters,
fluid
pools from your tears and
your sweat.
Your liquid self becomes
liquid for my home.
Forming in your image
I become you, and
You become me
A reflection in
the water of my womb.
No light, only dark
deep Primordial Waters.

Chapter 1

What to Expect

"Our invitation was accepted," my husband said, beaming with delight.

"Yes, it was," I whispered as my wide and tear-filled eyes looked at the tiny piece of plastic with the red line on it.

That moment of confirmation I was pregnant was an inflection point of a journey that started long before the pregnancy and one that would continue long after. Little did I know this soul that chose us as stewards of their development—and my womb as its gateway to life on Earth—would be as much my guide and teacher as I was to them.

We named this little spirit "Beamer" while in utero because it reflected our sense that we were blessed with a beam from the heavens. And for over three months her growing presence was our secret that we shared with only a few.

Everything about this experience was new. Out of fear that I would do something wrong and programming that dictated the expected steps to take, I waited until a medical professional confirmed the pregnancy before I let it be real. Through the years I would have a lot to learn about trusting my body and intuition. From the beginning, though, I held stubbornly to the sense this was a magical event, that the experience of being pregnant was aligned with a cosmic source of life and worked in harmony with it. I yearned for a community and a culture where ideas and conversation around the unspoken treasures of the unknown were normalized. Where pregnancy and motherhood were explored in that vein. I intuited that what I was seeking was out there, waiting to be found.

My intuition was affirmed, and it led me to some books that provided what I was craving. On my conception journey I found a wonderful book, called *The Conception Mandala: Creative Techniques for Inviting a Child Into Your Life*, by Mark Olsen and Samual Avital.

It is a small book that is loaded with thoughtful questions about what it means to bring a child into your family constellation. It was confronting and stirring to sit with questions about why we wanted a child and what we thought a child would bring us we didn't already have. We wrote an invitation for the soul we wanted to join us. We created a mandala that held our hopes and dreams. This was a far cry from books and experts with a scarcity and fear-based mentality.

Through my pregnancies, a few favorites included *The Pregnant Woman's Comfort Book*, by Jennifer Louden, and *Spiritual Midwifery,* by Ina May Gaskin. I also read books to keep me inspired and in a positive, affirming, and enlightened space. A book that stands out for me, one I have picked up a number of times throughout my life, is *A Woman's Worth*, by Marianne Williamson. Over the years, truly there have been lovely books and online resources created that are thoughtful and holistic.

Once I had medical confirmation of my pregnancy, the one book I could not wait to read was the famous and now infamous encyclopedia on pregnancy, *What to Expect When You're Expecting.*[1] I had given this book to many friends as a shower gift, and now it was finally my turn. I didn't want to wait for someone to give it to me, so I ventured out to Barnes & Noble to acquire my own. Given we had not shared the news of our conception, I remember a sort of stealthy feeling as I perused the pregnancy section of the store. This book, while new at the time of my pregnancy, is in its 5th edition and is self-proclaimed as America's pregnancy bible. For me it was an initiation. I became a member of an elite club. Whatever magic was on the pages of that book had meaning and significance *to me* because I had achieved the "pinnacle of womanhood"—getting pregnant.

When I cracked it open, I found page after page of everything negative I could expect during each month of my pregnancy. I was crushed. Was this something I was supposed to read and be supported by during my pregnancy? In my mind I quickly renamed it *What **Terrible** Things to Expect When You're Expecting* and tossed it on the shelf of our home office. Because my pregnancy experience was BG (before Google), it was handy to have as a reference manual. But even then, I knew it would give me the worst-case scenario surrounding my questions, so it got little use.

To be clear, I am not driving this point home to bash this book. It is the one I had experience with, and it reflects what I want to bring to light about motherhood in our current culture. This book and others like it are part of a system that, at its worst, supports a reductionist mentality and belief that women are reproductive machines that make babies, and at its best, provides up-to-date information on the physiological event of being pregnant. A machine needs an owner's manual. Masculine values and thinking lead us

---

1 In the 1995 edition, *What to Expect When You're Expecting* listed three authors: Arlene Eisenber, Heidi E. Murkoff, and Sandee E. Hathaway, RSN. The most current edition lists only Murkoff as author, so a contemporary citation of the book reads: Murkoff, Heidi. *What to Expect When You're Expecting.* Workman Publishing, 2016.

to believe there must be one "boss book" and that you only talk to the "experts" for the truth, and you don't look anywhere else.

What to Expect is a tribute to rescue culture. With so many things that can go wrong and so much need for expertise, the overall subtext of the book is that you will be overwhelmed, you will need rescuing, and you absolutely must follow the doctor's orders. This mindset doesn't live in a vacuum. To many people, this is the best thinking on this subject. It is the medicalization of motherhood, and it is the prevailing construct for moms.

It is also an excellent stand-in for the entire Mother Code because it is one very clear, concrete representation of the values one is meant to internalize. It would be more useful in an empowering context, and that's how we need to engage with a lot of the mainstream medical information that comes our way as the whole truth about mothering. No, it is not the whole truth, but it can have its place. But first *you* must find your place to know when and how you want to use it.

I took my dissatisfaction, as well as my hurt and anger, and I sought out books that were having a broader conversation. I wasn't seeking a watered-down or fanciful narrative; rather, one that would cause me to encounter myself, one that would invite me to go inside and see what is resonating and what isn't. I wanted to be fed, and I wanted nourishment that didn't stop at knowledge but ventured into the territory of wisdom and intuition. I yearned for a community of culture where ideas and conversation around the unspoken treasures of the unknown were normalized.

The years have passed, and now I find myself in the position of writing about motherhood in addition to reading about it. Yes, motherhood has been an amazing journey and continues to be so, but I want to make sure I don't fall into the point of view taken by many authors claiming to be *the* authority on motherhood. *What to Expect* fills a space in my own library, but I want to honor the many people who, through their own experience, research, and expansive thinking, have written about mothering in a capacious way.

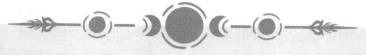

GROUNDING RITUAL

Use the earth's energy to support you and help you stay grounded as you navigate the myriad choices and decisions on the path of motherhood.

Plant your feet, sit on the earth, or imagine doing so in your mind's eye. Bring your awareness to the soles of your feet (or the base of your spine if sitting). Envision roots extending from these points, reaching down into the earth. With each breath, feel these roots growing deeper, anchoring you securely to the earth. Imagine the earth's energy, warm and nurturing, rising up through these roots, filling your body with a sense of stability and strength as you grow toward the light of the sun.

As you stand or sit, fully rooted, place your hands on your heart and silently affirm:

"I am grounded, steady, and supported by the earth beneath me."

Feel the energy of the earth flowing through you, giving you a deep sense of connection and support.

What Our Collective Future Can Look Like—And Yours

The experience of motherhood is driven by prevailing cultural beliefs and norms—many of which upend our footing and cause us to question our embodied reality. Challenges have always existed for mothers, but those challenges have been different depending on the period. Western culture is almost completely subsumed by

the hero myth, in which the masculine model of controlling, com-
partmentalizing, and mechanizing a natural process is a pretext
to "save" women from the pain of childbirth. We need to topple
the disempowering idea of pregnancy and birth as only a medical
event and return it to a sacred event where a woman reconnects
with her innate wisdom and is celebrated beyond her function to
produce a baby. We have been trained to avoid discomfort and to
fear pain. The good life is easy and pain-free. We crave comfort
and ease. The medical system offers practices to rid us of our pain.
It is synonymous with illness and death.

The center of our learning about our circumstance as a pregnant woman should be its sacrality, not worst-case scenarios. None
of the process should be desiccated, hidden, or made to be shame-
ful. We are trapped in a model where the wisdom encoded in a
woman's discomfort during pregnancy and pain during childbirth
are obscured by norms and practices that go unchecked. It is ironic
that during pregnancy we may wallow in suffering and victimhood, yet in birth we are shamed and ridiculed for uttering our
cries, when these cries call upon the intelligence that signals the
progressing stages of birth.

Mothering as a Synonym for Nurture

Mothering is nurturing. It is caring. It is all about the creative
and destructive forces we see in nature all around us all the time.
We are evolved beings, and for roughly the past 300,000 years
as Homo sapiens, we have been carrying out this experience.
And it is ever evolving and in our current day significantly more
complex and nuanced. At the same time, it is unchanging. Does
the weight of current complexities bear down on our predisposed
ability to nurture? Are women slotted into a role that says that
we are only here to nurture? Are we blocked by a masculine values paradigm that undervalues and takes for granted a powerful quality that is essential for our species to persist? It is so

confusing really. We are damned if we do (nurture) and damned if we don't (nurture)!

What does it mean to nurture? Why are women so wired for it? Is it natural, or is it something I am supposed to learn? It is natural, *and* we can feel cut off from this natural, innate part of us when it isn't valued. So, if you wonder why you aren't automatically plopped into nurture mode when your baby pops out, you are not broken, you need to reconnect and open up the pathways.

I remember being at dinner with one of my daughters and some friends of hers—all in their mid to late twenties. One of them mentioned that she and her husband were talking about starting a family. She expressed her fear that if she had a baby, she wouldn't love it as much as her mom had loved her when she was born. She said her mother often reveled in sharing how the minute she held her in her arms it was the best feeling in the world, and she just fell head over heels in love with her. My daughter turned to me and asked me if I felt the same way the minute *she* was born. My heart skipped a beat. I wanted to give her a different answer, but I told her the truth. I said that no, I did not experience the immediate "baby bliss" her friend's mom was describing. I felt guilty in that moment, as it had never hit me before that while I did feel like a goddess the moment she was born, it was more about me. I didn't want her to think I didn't love her, and while I didn't have it instantly, it came. That feeling built over time, but it took intention and work for me to open up to that shared experience.

I may have had the example of my loving grandparents, but my primary caregivers modeled a different, very transactional version of a relationship. Accessing deep feelings of love and affection for my children took time. For women who have had the experience of instantaneous love and connection, that is something to cherish. Those of us who did not, however, have nothing to be ashamed of. Just as I want you to understand that you have a deep reservoir of expertise and intelligence—in all meanings of that word—to draw on, I also want you to hear me when I say there is no right way to mother. If something does not come easily to you, that is not a sign of failure.

I spend my professional life working with moms, helping people grow into the parents they want to be. If I had not had the challenges in my own childhood and as a young mom I had, I would not be driven to do this work today. When we talk about nurturing our families, we must remember to nurture ourselves as well. That's how we grow into the people we yearn to be.

Motherhood Across Cultures

From a young age, we are made to believe that our culture's system of managing pregnancy, birth, and motherhood reflects steady improvement in humanity's understanding, our science, and our technology. As one begins to realize that the perspective of mothers is not prioritized or even respected during these vulnerable phases but instead managed and contained, this myth of progress begins to tatter around the edges. Is the best system one in which, once you learn about other cultures and how the ways we treat mothers has changed over time, the whole premise scatters like ashes in the wind?

We have—all of us—been programmed with a Mother Code that carries within it a whole set of assumptions and biases that turn being a mother into a profit center, one that gives mothers no more voice or choice than a consumer at a fast-food restaurant. But every society has its own version of the Mother Code. Understanding some differences can be important in learning how to rewrite our own Mother Code.

If we hopped in a time machine and set it for the Neolithic Era, roughly from 10,000 to 2,200 BCE, we would marvel at women and mothers occupying a central position in spiritual and social life. It seems that, of everything early humanity saw in the world, pregnancy and birth were holy and miraculous events. Reverence and honor were also held for women postmenopausal. Venus of

Willendorf, the 29,500-year-old figurine found in Austria, is often portrayed as a fertility symbol, when in actuality her features reflect a woman past her childbearing years.

Plenty of other evidence reinforces the idea that mothers were the beating heart of the communities in which they lived. Where later societies would use phallic symbols as a representation of strength, early society used vaginal symbols.[2] Psychologist and scholar Dr. Shari Thurer devoted years of her life to understanding the warp and woof of culture and its relationship to matriarchy across the millennia, and she has adroitly described the ins and outs of how that relationship has changed. As Thurer explains it, "...in many civilizations where the Goddess held sway, women did too, to a certain extent."[3] I am skeptical that our time machine could pinpoint a day and time in which everything shifted from an egalitarian culture to a patriarchal one, but the inquiry is valuable. All the theories have holes but Leonard Shlain put forth one that struck a chord with me in his book, *The Alphabet Versus the Goddess: The Conflict Between Word and Image*, where he lays out how the shifts in values coincided with the movement from oral storytelling and visual imagery to linear written language.

Patriarchy is not connected to a light switch; it doesn't turn on and off based on your understanding of it. We live in a society with deeply rooted, male-centered structures all around us. Moving toward a more balanced way of living will always be a work in progress. My husband and I agreed all along that we wanted to parent differently, in a way that was truer to who we are, and which focused on every family member's development. But that is the north star: You aim for it, it helps you navigate, but you don't judge your success on whether you have landed on the star.

---

2 Thurer, Shari. *The Myths of Motherhood: How Culture Reinvents the Good Mother*. Penguin, 1995, p. 9.

3 Thurer, p. 10.

In full transparency, despite a level of awareness that exceeded our parents, Rich and I still fell into traditional masculine and feminine roles. It would be years before I challenged these roles as my early zeal in mothering mindfully waned over time, and I began to recommit to a new path as a teacher and storyteller myself. Sometimes, it takes years of life experience before clouds lift and we see dysfunctional patterns and behaviors with more clarity.

Your journey in rewriting your own Mother Code will have these same fits and starts and transitions and seasons. What matters above all is the practice, the daily ritual of working to embrace your vision of your best self, and the best outcomes for your family in whatever season you are in.

The Mother and the Midwife

"Push!" my midwife directed me with a soft but firm tone. Seeing the look of terror on my face as I gripped the footboard of our bed, she grabbed my hands.

"Push into the pain," she said as she locked eyes with me.

"Is she nuts?" I thought. This was about the last thing I wanted to do. My brain was rejecting the invitation to intentionally move into the burning pain. But my trust in Mary overrode the desire to hold back and attempt retreating from the searing ring of fire I was experiencing as my baby was about to crown. And I did it!

"You have a daughter!" Kate and Mary said in unison.

What I remember most is those first moments was the energy that rippled through my body with the crystal-clear truth: "I AM A GODDESS!"

I love my midwives! There are not enough words for the gratitude I hold for them, not only for being there for the home births of both of our daughters, but also for being champions of keeping midwifery an option for all women. I watched as Mary fought tirelessly against a system that continues to layer challenge upon challenge, walling midwives off from providing services in general, and making it next to impossible for women who choose a birth outside of a hospital setting.

Mary poured herself into realizing one of her dreams when in 2014 she opened the first free-standing birth center in Illinois. Then in 2022, she started a fully accredited midwifery program for women from underrepresented communities in midwifery working toward birth equity and options for their communities. We have stayed closely connected and I work with her in her programs as adjunct faculty, where I have the privilege to support women striving for certification as doulas and midwives to mother themselves as they mother the mothers.

It infuriates me that the choice to birth with a midwife has become so difficult. We need not go back thousands of years to see the changing perceptions of birthing practices and how the Mother Code would have changed in kind. In the United States, women ruled over birth until relatively recent developments. Midwives delivered almost all babies in colonial times and continued to do so for many years. In the mid-1800s, male doctors took notice of these women-run medical events—as they perceived birth to be. They formed a lobby and documented marketing campaign to convince lawmakers and the public to curtail the use of midwives for deliveries so they could profit from what was suddenly viewed as a business.

Obstetricians in the U.S. were famously incompetent from the point of view of doctors in other countries. In 1910, Dr. Abraham Flexner published a long report[4] that extensively criticized American obstetricians and the schools where they were being trained. Flexner found the whole system so riddled with problems he recommended sending doctors to the U.K. for proper training and then returning them to the U.S.

---

4   A link to the full report can be found at http://archive.carnegiefoundation.org/publications/pdfs/elibrary/Carnegie_Flexner_Report.pdf.

Rather than seeing this as a wake-up call, American obstetricians reached that most self-centered of conclusions: To increase their reputation, and make more money, they would eliminate their competition: midwives. In 1912, shortly after Dr. Flexner's book was published, Professor J.W. Williams published a paper titled "Medical education and the midwife problem in the United States." In it, he argued for eliminating midwives, calling them dirty, untrained witches, and blaming them for maternal deaths.

Ironically, the data from this period indicates the exact opposite. Increased births in hospitals were leading to increases in mortality rates due to birth injuries by as much as *40-50%* between 1915 and 1929, according to one study. Another examined home births and hospital births between 1930 and 1932 and found that infant mortality in hospital births numbered 1.67 per 1,000, while home births had .90 infant deaths per 1,000 during that same period.[5] I am left feeling heartbroken and angry that the actual data was ignored and replaced with fraudulent and damaging propaganda.

Replacing the wisdom and woman-to-woman connection of a midwife was one of the so-called "advances" that included the development of the "twilight sleep." This was a method which employed a combination of the drugs scopolamine and morphine to make the delivering mother oblivious to what was happening. She would awaken after the birth with no memory of the event. This approach was combined with the crusade against midwives by prominent doctors of the period such as Dr. Joseph DeLee, who declared births dangerous and midwives incompetent.[6] Despite methods of pain relief having evolved in positive ways over the

---

5 This history is detailed in Thomasson, Melissa A., and Jaret Treber. "From home to hospital: The evolution of childbirth in the United States, 1928–1940." *Explorations in Economic History* 45.1 (2008): 76-99.

6 The Oregon Health & Science University has a brief and informative overview of the history of midwives in the U.S. in the 20th century on its website, ohsu.edu under https://www.ohsu.edu/womens-health/brief-history-midwifery-america

years, doctors remain at the highest elevation of esteem with midwives operating on the fringes of birth in America.

The forces of this ardent intention of the male-dominated medical establishment to rule over conception, pregnancy, and birth have woven their way so completely into our mainstream culture most women are blind to its malintent. Even as a white, cis woman with a great deal of privilege, I could feel the constraint the nurse midwives were under to provide a home birth. I was surprised to discover that a home birth was significantly less expensive than a hospital birth. Yes, that hospital cost would mostly be covered by insurance, but let's not ignore the obvious benefit of the hospital-insurance business relationship that would have a lot to lose if they started including home birth.

It made sense that our midwives were required to partner with a MD in a hospital as a backup if I needed to transfer to a hospital. But what doesn't make sense is how difficult it is to find doctors who will do it—in part because of both the perceived risk and making less money, but mostly because of the stigma of being part of what is now considered a rogue practice.

We had one meeting with our backup doc, aptly named Dr. Angela, and she was lovely. It was comforting to know that the woman who would receive us in the hospital if needed was an advocate of home birth and that she concluded by saying she hoped to *not* see us again! Looking back on it now, what stands out for me was the sense of aloneness on Dr. Angela's part. She may not have said it directly, but I was left with a foreboding feeling like an animal on the brink of extinction.

What women of all backgrounds had been accomplishing without medical apparatus for millennia is now viewed as beyond the grasp of most women once men had control over what became and remains the business of birth.

Mothering the Mother

Across the globe, rest for mother is deeply embedded in tradition. In Mexico, it is known as *cuarentena*. The Chinese phrase for it is translated into "doing the month." The Japanese call it *satogaeri bunben*, and women traditionally return home to their parents for this period. In Eastern Europe, there is typically a one-month period of seclusion following birth. In Latin America, a period of seclusion is accompanied with body massage to aid recovery.[7] If we examine contemporary practices across cultures spanning the globe, we see a pattern of support for mothers after birth that isn't reflected here in the United States.

Generally, the consensus in other countries seems to be that, for at least 40 days after birth, mothers must rest and be given special consideration. That can be support from others (especially other women), a particular diet, isolation, and lots of rest.[8] The specifics vary, but this practice of support is so common that its absence in American culture is notable.

Northern European nations' respect for mothers after birth is codified into law. In the Netherlands, every mother receives a *kraamzorg*, or maternity carer, following birth, usually for eight days.[9] Finland sends every mother a "maternity package" with 63 essentials for the newborn in a box that can be a bed for the baby. Antenatal care is standard and free for mothers in these countries. The U.S. follows no such tradition and has no federal provisions for family medical leave.[10] Our go-it-alone society has

---

7 Healthline has a very good overview of these global practices and traditions at https://www.healthline.com/health/pregnancy/what-post-childbirth-care-looks-like-around-the-world-and-why-the-u-s-is-missing-the-mark.

8 These practices are enumerated in: Eberhard-Gran, Malin, et al. "Postnatal care: a cross-cultural and historical perspective." *Archives of Women's Mental Health* 13 (2010): 459-466.

9 The Guardian website at guardian.com has an article about this titled "A home help for eight days after giving birth? Why Dutch maternity care is the envy of the world." The link is https://www.theguardian.com/lifeandstyle/2023/oct/25/a-home-help-for-eight-days-after-giving-birth-why-dutch-maternity-care-is-the-envy-of-the-world.

10 The website annuity.com publishes data on maternity leave by state. As of this writing, the most current year available on the site was 2023 and can be found at https://www.annuity.org/personal-finance/financial-wellness/average-paid-maternity-leave-by-state/.

engineered a family structure which for decades encouraged the idea of a family including two parents and their children and then left mom to fend for herself following births.[11] I don't know about you, but this is mind-boggling and heartbreaking that a country that proclaims to be one of the most advanced in the world is the only *developed* country on the planet to neglect to provide for its children and families.

Cultural context matters. What seems fixed and certain in our society can be a relatively new innovation. Mothers should define and design the Mother Code through which we all see this essential identity. Michelle Walks and Naomi McPherson's ambitious *An Anthropology of Mothering* provides tremendous cultural and historical context and brings the topic back to the core of its importance. They write, "*mothering* is about behavior, practices, and engagement...*mothering* is about biology *and* culture, bodies *and* being...*mothering* is practiced by more than just *mothers.*"[12] By articulating mothering in this holistic way, a vision emerges that expands beyond a singular role or narrow identity.

We Are All Mothers

Mothering others is a beautiful offering from which many women derive pleasure, satisfaction, and meaning. The imperative of valuing our service to others as a gift rather than an expectation falls on us. The more *we* claim the value of our caring labor, the more it will be reflected back to us and the disparity that exists will come into balance.

We ALL mother, with or without children. We conceive, create, and give birth to children, relationships, careers, pets, dreams, and frankly anything we put our caring, nurturing, protective energy into. You will hear this expressed as a drumbeat throughout the

---

11 You can read a history of family structure's midcentury development at https://online. csp.edu/resources/article/the-evolution-of-american-family-structure/.

12 Walks, Michelle, and Naomi McPherson. *An Anthropology of Mothering*. Demeter Press, 2011, 9.

book. We must hear paradigm-shifting concepts many times before we take notice. Claiming the mother identity as an inherent part of your existence only empowers you. Giving birth is not the golden ticket that gets you into an elite club. Rather, it is a choice you make on how you want to use your creative power and spend your precious energy. A child is one of many paths a mother can take.

In my workshops, I invite people to introduce themselves like this: "My name is (fill in name), and I am a mother." Because of our programming, this simple act of naming what is true evokes a full range of emotions and reactions for people without a child under their care. I have seen on their faces and heard in their voices everything from joy to pain to anger. I have seen relief, discomfort, and outright refusal to utter these words. I understand how it feels sacrilegious and scandalous to make what some would consider a false claim on an identity that we have been programmed to believe we must earn or can only achieve by giving birth or raising a child. I have even had stepmothers tell me they were shamed or criticized for calling themselves a mother if they didn't give birth to the child that they are now responsible for raising.

It is essential that we find common ground among each other and foster genuine sisterhood. If we want to connect with divine mother energy and our creative power and put it to good use in the world, we must adopt an inclusive mindset that inspires us to see the myriad ways we all mother. And, that we acknowledge all the ways in which we have been a mother. If you have set your path on motherhood, you may feel fear and trepidation about this new endeavor; and that is expected. But I also invite you to consider all the ways you have been a mother in so many other areas of your life.

If you have cared about someone or something, you have mothered. If you have put time and energy and passion into creating something, you have mothered. If you have experienced heartache at the loss of someone meaningful, you have mothered.

As you nurture this new neural wiring, it will let you build on your experiences with the wisdom and knowledge you have accumulated on your journey. Then consider the ways you will learn, grow, and develop during motherhood, all the while building the next layer of your becoming. This cycle ultimately leads you back to mothering in other ways than children again. You come full circle!

Mothering Careers

I consider it a privilege to have so many women in my universe that have chosen to put their mother energy into their careers—both with and without children. Some I have coached directly and others I am close to as friends, so I have intimate knowledge of their journey.

It was during my original doctoral workshop, which only included women without children in their care, when I first shared the idea that all women mother. I thought this was an important but tangential piece I was including. The main intention of the workshop was to raise their awareness and open the door for them to critically discern all the choices they would face to prepare for motherhood—and throughout motherhood. But after I dropped in the piece that they were already mothers, and that they have been mothering in many ways in their lives, it hit me. I realized just how harsh and limiting the programming that dictates nothing you achieve or accomplish in your life is as important or meaningful than having a child.

It broke my heart to hear one of the participants share that despite having created a highly successful interior design and build agency, she felt none of it ultimately mattered and she was a failure if she didn't also get married and have a child.

When I was in the beginning stages of my desire to take my doctoral work out to the world, I engaged a woman-owned personal branding agency to help me put words to what I was doing. To my delight, Jessica, the founder of the agency, had a dream in which she was given the words I use today—the Mother Code. I owe her my sincere gratitude for this. As I worked with her, I also did some private coaching for her personally. Jessica still questioned whether she wanted to be a mother of children in her life, yet she did the beautiful work owning and celebrating the mother energy she was already putting into creating her business. Everyone around her, including her husband and employees, could feel the shift.

When she shared her excitement about this new revelation on her social media platform, a friend reached out very upset. She told Jessica she had no right to claim being a mother if she didn't have children. She chose to hold her ground and share with her friend what this meant to her. Jessica said while she was not claiming they were the same experiences, owning her mother energy and identifying as a mother was real and very much alive and present for her. She mothered herself powerfully both by claiming her identity on the mother continuum and guarding it when it was questioned.

Whether you are an entrepreneur, an employee, part of a team, a CEO, or anywhere you must take care of people or a project, you are mothering.

It is so beautiful and empowering when we recognize the mother energy we provide in these endeavors. When we do, we see the parallel cycle of conceiving, creating, and birthing that most endeavors require.

Mothering Relationships

Relationships also require mothering. No matter what the pairing looks like from a gender perspective, healthy relationships thrive when mother energy is present. (They need father energy also, but that is a topic of another book!) The parallel I want to shine the light on is that like children are our mirrors that stir up the "unfinished business" from our formative years, our partners and closest relationships do the same thing. How we were mothered in our upbringing shows up in every relationship. It is not *if* you will be triggered it's *when*, and how will you deal with it.

Elsa, a woman who exudes a fierce mother love endowed from her Icelandic heritage, and her husband Corrado, a feisty and strong-willed Italian, make a powerful couple. But what makes them a thriving couple is their dedication to continuously learning and growing, working on their relationship, and supporting others to do the same. What inspires me about them is that while my husband and I focused our collective energy into parenting our children and stopped vibrantly growing, this couple turned up the volume. Yes, they parented their twins thoughtfully, but they didn't lose themselves in the chaos to do it.

So even if children do not put demands on a long-term relationship, without a powerful vision and consciousness toward activating it and keeping alive the values you mutually share, the chances of its failing increase exponentially. Relationships need care and feeding and vigilance to keep growing and evolving. Sounds like mothering!

Mothering the Unexpected

Sometimes, children or people come in and out of our lives in very unexpected ways. Sometimes, the child we expected or dreamed of is not the child we receive into our care. From my perspective, these circumstances surrounding the unexpected have what would generally be considered a tragedy or loss attached to them. You give birth to a beautiful baby only to discover they have an incurable disease. Or, because of the death of their mother and father, a child enters your life as you were named their chosen guardian. Life throws us so many twists and turns, and the life we envisioned, or more accurately the life we are programmed to envision, as the "good" life can go off the rails when it doesn't fit our picture.

I want to honor all the women who have experienced the loss of a child at any stage. Whether it was through a terminated pregnancy, a miscarriage, or a stillbirth, the loss is acute and intense. Our culture has little to no support or tolerance for this loss and you are expected to bounce back and get back on your feet without enough time and space to grieve. You mothered a little soul even if it was for a few weeks or months. Whatever the circumstances for their short life—and death—cycle, it affected you; and there is much to mine from it as an experience of mothering yourself and another.

I also want to acknowledge those whose mothering experience was outside normal parameters.

When my brother and sister-in-law had their second child, a son, they soon noticed delays and behavioral issues. But it would take years and incredible determination on their part to accurately diagnose Phelan-McDermid syndrome (pronounced FAY-luhn mick-DUR-mid). PDS is a rare genetic disorder involving chromosome 22 that can affect many critical functions in a person's body—from learning and communicating to eating and sleeping.

Their son is now 18, and I was recently with them to celebrate his sister's college graduation. During the weekend, I experienced so many emotions, and my realizations were unexpected. On the first night together, all I could think about was how glad I was that we were not dealt this hand. Imagine for a moment the time and energy required to care for a toddler, the vigilance of attention and sleep deprivation, as your forever parenting reality. How did they do it? How are they not just a jumble of nerves and puddles of resentment pooling on the floor? In all honesty, what I was harboring was pity for them—"Oh my poor brother, sister-in-law, and niece—they sure got the short end of the stick" was what kept running through my mind.

By the end of the next day my judgment of this being a "hard" situation started to melt. Yes, it is full of challenges above and beyond what a typical family navigates during their children's lives, but here they were, rolling with it. They were having distance and humor and going about their lives as we all do. I can't tell you how they have done what is heroic, but I can say what I felt and what I saw them orient to was nothing other than L-O-V-E, love!

What I witnessed was not just any kind of love, but pure unconditional love in action. I didn't feel victimhood or sacrifice or hardship because to them it's simply loving their special-needs son as they do their daughter. People talk about love all the time but little of what we give, or experience, is unconditional. That is a part of mother love. When there is no reciprocation, no affirmation, or gratitude for what you are doing for someone, it must be something as powerful as love that sustains you.

Women mother under any circumstances. Grieving the loss of what you had imagined or assumed would be your motherhood reality is part of your journey and should be honored. Our capacity for love and caring is infinite in its forms and endurance.

Mothering the Aged

Many of us face or will encounter the reality of aging parents, other family members, or friends who need mothering. The global pandemic highlighting this as the care gap was put in high relief. Women are the default caregivers. We cannot help ourselves! I don't have a problem with this as I honor how it is second nature for us to jump in and fill the holes. I take issue when this laboring is undervalued and underappreciated. We will continue to do it anyway, but the cost to ourselves and the world needs to be recognized because were it to be given adequate acknowledgment through tangible (an abundant wage) and intangible (a heartfelt thank you) ways, there would only be more of it available, as we would be sustained. And truly, our world needs more mother energy. The need for our care is ever-present and shows up in many ways, another of which is caring for the aging.

In 2019, a writer published an anonymous piece on Lesley Jane Seymour's Covery Club website, which is geared toward topics of interest to middle-aged women. The piece was titled "When

A Good Daughter Hates Caring for Her Aging Mother."[13] The daughter in the title was the writer. She complained about caring for her 92-year-old mother and about the shame she felt for resenting her. It was a relatively short but very honest essay.

Hundreds of comments thanked her profusely for saying what many were feeling. "This is me," one comment began. "Your article was 'spot on,'" another said. The commentators were, overwhelmingly, the middle-aged women for whom the site was developed, and they were describing the heartbreaking struggle so many women face and, often, the anger they felt because they had to face it alone.

I can definitely relate.

Because of both ageism and the fears (reminders that death is close by) that surround aging, our Western American culture often chooses to shut elderly parents away. This can occur by putting them in a home, turning the care over to others, walking away, or shutting them out emotionally. I had done them all and was content with the feeling that my obligation ended with my financial contribution to my mother's care and occasional visits and excursions. I am not admonishing myself or putting myself in bad daughter prison. But I am acknowledging that it took making a conscious choice to step out of the boundaries I'd put between us while I was individuating and breaking our pattern of enmeshment.

These parameters were the best way I knew at the time to take care of myself around her borderline personality and narcissistic tendencies. Once I made this choice and decided to shine light on how I was past needing the same boundaries, beautiful gifts were revealed.

The first gift was laying down the resentment and belief that my mother's words or behavior still held the same power they did when I was a child. I chose to experience her as a quirky old lady who says mean and judgmental things sometimes, but also has a huge caring heart and resilience like no one I know. It was that

---

13 For those who are struggling with a similar situation, it's worth a read. You can find it at https://www.coveyclub.com/blog_posts/daughter-hates-caring-aging-mother/.

easy. I was no longer a victim to my mother, and the self-protective measures I once needed to give me space to develop a core sense of myself were no longer required. I didn't tell her I was doing this, but it didn't take her long to pick up on it and let me know how much she appreciated me letting her in. She didn't punish me or criticize my past behavior; rather, she acknowledged the necessity of it and was so glad for this new chapter of our relationship.

The second gift centers on my expanding compassion for and acceptance of the aging process. Our culture has an unhealthy relationship with the natural process of aging. Women are held to completely impractical and impossible goals of looking like you do in your 20s when you are 80. It is absurd and physically and emotionally violent to us to be pushed into this trap. I go there despite my best efforts to be above it and not care about the wrinkles and sagging everything. Part of the care for my mother involves seeing her naked 94-year-old body; and to be honest, it used to make me feel frightened and disgusted.

As I have worked to become more compassionate toward my own aging body, I view her body as natural and beautiful the way the Grand Canyon is magnificent. It is the reflection of time spent on this planet and the wounds of nature scaring the landscape that evoke awe in its beholders. Our bodies mirror this miracle, and even when I struggle to *love* my postmenopausal body, I can start by accepting it. If I had not chosen to drop my guard and tune into my caring and unconditional positive regard for my mother, I would have missed out on these precious gifts.

I hope these examples of mothering in its innumerable manifestations show the ways you are bringing your creative and caring energy to bear. And whether it affirms you, inspires you, or enlightens you, there is no question that you are a mother. You are a woman on her journey, amassing mothering experiences and sharing her gifts in gorgeous ways.

Crafting New Expectations

The ability of women to access our emotional intelligence and intuition is so powerful that it has been spun as a liability by people who seek to control us. "Overly emotional woman" has become such a central myth in our marginalization that it appears everywhere in our culture. Although the great intellects and artists across centuries—women and men—have affirmed the value of emotions and intuition in their pursuits of knowledge and art, the rest of us are left feeling a little disadvantaged when we recognize strong feelings in a room or react with emotion to a stirring sight or sound.

Once and for all: The intelligence of women is the intelligence of a loving universe! They are the same. Not using one's emotional awareness or intuitive sense when trying to sort out a problem is like tying one hand behind your back. If we're trying to solve the world's problems, if we're trying to make the planet more livable for everyone (and everything), then why wouldn't we use the full range of our intelligence to do these things? The answer may be in the question. If your goal is to make money or dominate others, those with a more holistic view can be threatening to your agenda.

The mainstream cultural perspective of modern society, its zeitgeist, is obviously blinkered, and we are setting the planet afire and subjecting billions to misery because of it. So, let's talk for a minute about full women's intelligence—in particular, emotions—and what unlocking it can do for you. Always remember: As you heal yourself, as your grow yourself, you grow, heal, and nurture the planet, and simply by diving into these topics, you are transforming the whole world.

The time with your conception, pregnancy, birth, and new motherhood is precious and fleeting. You don't have the energy, nor should you, to put it into navigating the voices of so many experts or your friends and family telling you how to mother. You are at your rawest and most vulnerable and your emotional labor needs to be spent wisely. The experience is a roller coaster of emotions, with many big and small feelings which can feel out of control.

An aspect of this time is truly chaos and disruption. Just as storms, fires, volcanos, and earthquakes are powerful events of disequilibrium and destruction in nature, they are also part of natural transformational cycles of our Earth. They cleanse, renew, and precipitate new growth and development. The same is true of our mothering journey. Pregnancy rocks our world like an earthquake with everything inside shifting and making room for its guest. We start to realize that we have little control over the physical experience. Birth is a volcanic eruption where new life emerges from our core. In drawing these parallels with nature's tumultuous yet transformative events, we understand that the experience of birth and mothering is about physical changes and a profound reorientation of our being.

What if you had moments where you could peek out from behind the curtain of the tumult, uncertainty, and monotony of new motherhood? What would you see? What if you opened yourself to the rhythms of nature, and tapped into the profound sacredness of this natural and mystical time? When you tune into your voice, it brings you into the present moment and that is where magic and all sorts of wonder become possible. Consider the following possibilities...

Conception is a surrender into the unknown.
Pregnancy is an expansion of self.
Birth is a portal connecting us with divine mystical energy.
New motherhood is reciprocal love in action.

Now, resonate with the above assertions. What feelings arise as you read or say them aloud? This is an invitation to not just understand these declarations but to feel them, to let them reverberate within you. It may feel challenging to some, or it may rekindle a spark of inner knowing for others. These emotions stirring— whether fear, anger, sadness, joy, or a blend of them all—are valid. The key is to stay open and curious.

Declarations such as the ones I offered here are the reflections of truths buried deep in the far reaches of our consciousness. They are the echo of our prepatriarchal mothers, grandmothers, and what some may call the goddess, or what Viki Noble refers to in her book, *Motherpeace: A Way to the Goddess Through Myth, Art, and Tarot*, as "the lost parent of humankind."[14] This is the fecundity of the universe reverberating through the oldest parts of our sentience.

We don't even know to yearn for this way of being, let alone consider surrendering to it. Instead, we robotically follow a script programmed into us by our family and culture where the most we ask for is a good night's sleep and the health and safety of our child. I am not knocking either thing; and I am especially not reducing the importance of a child's health and safety or the devastation at the loss of a child. I am acutely aware that in the United States there are a disproportionate number of parents and mothers, particularly mothers of color, where basic needs are at a premium and who struggle daily for survival.

This is all the more reason for women at any level of privilege to create a culture that both honors and engages in life from a mother-centered framework. One where the health and the well-being (physically, emotionally, and spiritually) of *both* mother and child are held in reverence and given every means of support to thrive. When we do the work to free ourselves from the shackles of a masculine-dominant culture and claim our personal freedom, we have the power to forge a path toward much needed equanimity among all people who mother.

---

14 Noble, Vicki. *Motherpeace: A Way to the Goddess Through Myth, Art, and Tarot.* Harper & Row, 1983.

Another way of seeing and living is within our grasp. The truths I describe as buried are also connected to our consciousnesses by a silver thread of embedded awareness. This thread connects to the brain beginning at the moment of conception. A woman's body transforms through pregnancy; the transformations of the mother's brain are less well-known, but they are just as real and just as profound. I am inviting you on an exploration through this book, but I am also telling you, you have taken the first steps, that your entire being is ready for this transformation—and was, in a deep and cosmic way. It's been ready since before you were born.

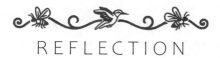

REFLECTION

Connect again with the energy of earth as you explore the ground you traversed in this chapter. Let Mother Earth hold you as you sift through thoughts and reactions you are having. You can also release any emotions that have built up inside into you; Mother Earth will absorb them and use it as fertilizer for new growth.

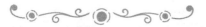

It's true. Conception, pregnancy, birth, new motherhood, childlessness…are all messy, painful, and difficult. So what? Some parts are naturally hard because our existence as an evolved species is based on enduring challenging circumstances. Evolution demands a high price. It is also hard because we live in a culture that doesn't recognize or honor a woman's natural capacities and gifts.

But when we put all of that to the side, we see that the process is simple really. When we choose to have a child as part of our mothering journey, we can expect to be part of an elegant physiological event that has been billions of years in the making. We can think as practical or as deep as we want. It doesn't matter because through all the advances and setbacks in evolution, natural or human created, we will still conceive, create, birth, and raise babies.

We can experience the physical changes our body goes through from a place of fear and dread and something we can't wait to get over with. We can experience it like visiting a new and foreign country. In that strange and novel place, I am uncomfortable with all the differences and lack of conveniences I am used to. Rather than complain and suffer, I can sit in the sheer awe and wonder of growing a human inside of my body, or watching my child accomplish something—from pooping to walking.

As women, we expect to encounter many opinions, expert advice, and media images that both support our highest potential in mothering as well as tear it down and make it needlessly difficult. But we have the power to remember how wondrous it is that we have a brain, emotional facility, generational legacy, and a spiritual knowing that lets us choose what voices we listen to and resonate with.

We've come to expect judgment, reactions, and feelings about our choices as women. But we can recognize it all as reflections of a population that's been disconnected from our mothering, feminine energy and has lost the core sense of ourselves. Let's also remember that our greatest capacity as humans is to nurture and care about not only our children but our friend's child, our sister's child, our neighbor's child, and children in other countries—all children *and* most important the mothers of those children.

Evolution has gifted us with highly evolved brains that have the capacity to navigate this territory in such profoundly elevated, passionate, pleasurable, and soul-expanding ways. Even the most glancing, brief experience of this realm of awareness is worth the work you put into it. While women have struggled a lot across the millennia, there has not been a steady unbroken history of men calling the shots, especially regarding pregnancy and birth.

The future need not be defined exclusively by what has become tragically familiar—and it shouldn't be.

Chapter 2

Understanding the Mother Code

When people hear "Rewrite the Mother Code," they ask me, "What?! What does that mean?" It means a lot! It means so many things. It encapsulates both experiences in raising children and the mothering we do in all facets of our life.

Rewriting the Mother Code is unique to the individual. It means choosing what works best for your life rather than living by societal, cultural, or familial norms. It's not about abandoning all you have known or done before but intentionally curating a meaningful and fulfilling life. Here's one way to describe it: Rewriting the Mother Code is a way to profoundly shape your experience as a mother by identifying limiting internal and external ideas about how you should be, and replacing them with mindsets that promote your self-worth and your capacity for personal development. At the same time, you are strengthening your capacity to mother in the most loving and effective way possible.

And that is only the beginning! Rewriting your Mother Code is a pathway on the journey of coming home to the self that knows you are and always have been a mother. It activates your deep knowing you are and always will be loved unconditionally as a daughter of Mother Universe. You will reawaken, discover, and heal lost parts of yourself and find wholeness in your being.

Uncover. Explore. Both within yourselves and in your cultures, families, and surroundings. What does doing motherhood differently look like to you? What will you be up against? Bring more awareness of the choices you can make. Tune into yourself, your intuition, and your body. What does it feel like in your body? It might not make sense to anyone else. But it makes sense to you. Be the mother in your life. Claim that. Consciously choose and envision an ideal state.

I recommend applying that approach in many areas of your life. For example, this book is written using the philosophy of the Rewritten Mother Code. I am speaking to head and heart, to you as a woman and as a child of the cosmos. This is not your mother's mothering book! On the one hand, it is much more complex and nuanced, simply because it is written from a matricentric view that challenges ideas in this country that have reigned dominant for only a generation. On the other, it is not complicated for the sake of it. I am convinced that by illuminating the layers—and seeing the manifold meanings of motherhood (including mothering children)—the benefit will be exponentially more impactful.

In doing so, I hope to speak to all women, people who have chosen to have children, and those not willing or able to have kids. All are invited to connect to the mothering experience. I will show you how to plug into the mother energy and the powerful rhythms of the conceive, create, give birth, and raise children cycle through which we are all wired. You'll learn to use it all to your benefit in so many impactful ways. The Mother Code bridges the gap between women with and without children and honors all of our choices.

I also wish to serve the woman initially inviting a child into her life. This idea provides a framework for navigating her choices surrounding conception and making those choices consciously while learning and growing through the whole spectrum of motherhood. This woman wants to do it differently and more mindfully than the current norm dictates.

For the new mom who is scared because she is experiencing something she wasn't expecting (positive or negative) and wants to get back on track for a more growth-focused, nourishing experience, I am honored to meet you on that journey. As a newly pregnant woman, you may be feeling excited and hungry to explore possibilities for this new chapter of your life—welcome.

All too often, the mother launching her children into the world is kept out of the conversation. I wish to celebrate the mom with older children on the precipice of a new phase and those in the next phase of life without children. I trust we will see the intersection of this woman with the women who remained childfree. While she may have adult children to navigate, her life is fully hers, and she is curious about how she wants to mother now.

Wherever you sit on your mothering journey, you probably have an inkling, or are experiencing, that all is not well in the *motherland*! You may be feeling hurt and angry because of the internalized expectations put on you from your family or culture telling you how to mother. You may also be wondering how to do this mothering thing *right* or what *right* even means. Maybe you don't always like what you see around you, and how you've been living isn't what you want, but you don't know how to change it. You may also feel hopeful because you sense there is a different way to mother and you're ready to explore possibilities for creating a mothering experience that is your own.

The opportunity outlined in this book of a mothering experience that transcends the overwhelm, self-sacrifice, and self-doubt that proliferates in our current mothering culture comes from my lived experience and from the women I coach and surround myself with. I have been in all the places—days filled with doubt and fear; trying to do it right; meltdowns... I have also experienced incredible personal healing and transformation. I am proud of ways my husband and I parented consciously with self-awareness and emotional intelligence. I intend to honor the full experience, from fear and doubt, to self-aware and present.

If I find I'm self-blaming for what I didn't know or information I didn't have access to, I allow myself to look at the wider picture. My goal is that, on a person-to-person level, the current mothering culture fails fewer women in the future. This is what I am working to change. I intend that my contribution for the remaining decades of my life creates an archetype where the feminine values, reverence, and support absent in our current culture become the norm. Together we can bring about a league of women and husband/partner allies in a way that I did not experience but I know is possible.

The world needs a lot more mother! The world needs a transfusion of this particular kind of love right now. We need to give ourselves this love first and foremost and then share it with everyone and everything we put our caring energy into. The beauty of, and my hope for, having these coexist is that all the stories serve each woman in their own personal way as well and bring them together in a community of awareness.

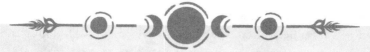

BREATH RITUAL

Breath is life force energy. It connects us to ourselves and to everything that breathes on this planet. Our breath is the loving mother energy that provides us strength and power.

Tune into your breathing. Notice where your breath naturally flows—does it come from your chest, your belly, or somewhere else? Recognize that your breath is a mirror, reflecting your current emotional and physical state. This awareness is the foundation of the ritual, grounding you in the present moment.

Play with different kinds of breath, as each has the power to provide what you need as you mother...

Breath of Fire: Breathe fast and hard from your chest in a continuous flow for ten seconds. Focus on the rapid rise and fall of your chest as you energize your body with this breath. After completing the cycle, place your hands over your heart and say aloud or silently, "Breath of fire, I honor you for providing me with bursts of energy in a moment of need. You fuel my passion and drive, and I am grateful." Notice how your body feels after this breath. Are you energized? How has your emotional state shifted? Allow yourself to experience the sensations that arise.

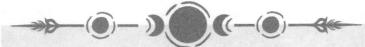

Sustaining Breath: Inhale slowly and deeply into your belly, placing your hands on your abdomen to feel it rise like a balloon. Exhale slowly, feeling your belly soften with the release of air. With your hands still on your belly, express your gratitude by saying, "Thank you, sustaining breath, for your healing and calming rhythms. You ground me, nourish me, and bring me peace." Savor the sense of calm and stability that this breath brings, noticing any shifts in your emotional state or physical body. Embrace the stillness that follows.

Ocean Breath (Ujjayi Breath): Breathe deeply through your nose with a slight constriction in the back of your throat, creating a soft oceanic sound. This breath can be deeply calming and centering. As you breathe, affirm, "Ocean breath, I thank you for your soothing waves that wash over me, bringing clarity and peace."

As you conclude the ritual, return to your natural breath. Notice any changes in your emotional state, energy levels, and physical sensations. Offer a final affirmation of gratitude: "Thank you, breath, for being my constant companion. I honor you as the bridge between my body, mind, and spirit."

Carry the awareness of your breath with you as you go about your day, remembering it is always available to guide, support, and strengthen you.

What Is the Mother Code?

From the moment you discover you have conceived a child, or you have recognized your own maternal powers, you enter a season of your life that eclipses all experiences that have come before it. Whether your conception experience involves receiving a child through adoption or foster care, step-parenthood, guardianship, or otherwise, there are many possibilities. It could be filled with challenges, or be simple and straightforward, planned, or an unexpected turn of events. Despite the varying degrees of experiences, one thing is a constant: You are forever changed. Whether that cosmic life force that chose you as a steward for its entry into this world stays with you for days, months, or a lifetime, you have the power inside you to choose the mothering experience that resonates with your deepest desires. That is the beauty, the power, and the potential that lies in motherhood. Even if you have some trepidation (or terror!) about the journey ahead, something inside of you, some still small voice, knows this to be true.

Sadly, our current Western American culture is filled with messages and challenges that too often silence your intuitive voice and veer us away from exploring a person-centered motherhood experience. Also, family culture, and the wiring laid down in our formative years, becomes our scripted voice. These messages from our family and culture are the Mother Code. Any restrictive, disempowering, or unexamined belief, process, or expected behavior in your mothering journey is considered a Mother Code. I discourage you from labeling them good or bad and instead hold a nondualistic approach. What you seek outside of the consensual reality of the Mother Code may be labeled unconventional, or even dangerous.

In hindsight, it is clear what messages I chose to listen to, and when. Sometimes I even knew in the moment I was going against my intuition or gut sense of something. I felt a sense of fear I was making choices not in alignment with my values or my sense of what was right for me—even if it wasn't logical. How is it we come to make the choices we make on our mothering journey? What factors and circumstances impact our choices, consciously and unconsciously?

Your Childhood Code

You are a sponge! Yep, you are an adorable sponge soaking up everything. You are taking it all in. You feel the vibes from the atmosphere you are conceived in. You hear sounds from within your womb home. You share the experience of birth with your mother. You are raw material. You are vulnerable, helpless, and eager to absorb everything in your surroundings. You feel EVERYTHING! You feel the waves of joy or terror or sadness that ripple through your mother's body when she discovers you are growing inside of her. You feel both the love and the tentativeness of her embrace.

Beyond the DNA of your lineage, which is preset, additional wiring is happening every second of your new existence. In the primal dance of relationship with your closest caregivers, you begin to interpret their moods, behaviors, and responses. You respond in ways you hope ensures your continued survival.

In this liminal time that precedes explicit memory, you are building core beliefs about yourself, the world outside of you, what you can expect from the world, and what the world can expect from you. In an ideal scenario, we would emerge from childhood with a solid sense we matter and we are loved. We would believe the world is a safe place for us to learn, grow, and make mistakes. We are seen and see others. We are supported and support others. On the other end of the spectrum, we can also form a belief that we don't exist. We may be consumed with thoughts like, *I am too much. I am not enough. The world is a dangerous place and does not want the best for me. I will hoard my resources lest I be taken advantage of.* We may have a mix of these or show up anywhere on the continuum.

Studies show that whatever the results of your relationship dance, the beliefs you form are wired in by roughly two years of age. Being the brilliant beings that we are, we then build behaviors or coping mechanisms that continue to affirm the original beliefs, and in our best little-self ways, we try to meet our hunger to be seen and heard—even if that attention is negative.

The foundation of our own mothering experiences at its best is a product of reflection, not reaction, regardless of the mothering experience we had as children and our reaction to it. Without self-awareness or exploration, we will unconsciously do what we experienced, or, on the flip side, we swing the pendulum and go in the exact opposite direction.[1] Being in reflection lets us be intentional about making our own choices. Even if we had a wonderful experience, we still want to question the choices our mothers made so we make the exploration of mothering our own. And we want to learn from, rather than react to, the challenging experiences of growing up.

Something I am most proud of in my life is my dedication to the exploration and rewriting of my childhood codes. Diving into those depths of feeling, expressing, healing, and understanding has been a lifelong quest that will never be complete until I die, and even then, my spirit will continue its evolution. As described by sociologist Jack Mezirow across his body of work, our childhoods are responsible for our *formation,* then as adults we have the choice to use that experience for our *transformation.* As I share my story, I invite you to ride alongside me so you can tell your story that reveals the Mother Codes you formed in your childhood.

My mother's womb and birth canal—my home and pathway into this world—reverberated with the echoes of deeply painful and harrowing experiences from her past. The first trauma experienced by my mother, that I am aware of, happened when she was around 21 years old. It was an abortion at the hands of underground

---

1 This phenomenon is explained in detail in Daines, Chantel L., et al. "Effects of Positive and Negative Childhood Experiences on Adult Family Health." *BMC Public Health* 21 (2021): 1-8.

practitioners—which sadly they all were in the 1950s. As if this wasn't traumatic enough, the police busted the place while she was recovering from her abortion. Shortly after her procedure, the officers escorted my mother home to her surprised, but fortunately compassionate, parents.

A couple years later, my mother was the victim of nonconsensual sex (her words not mine, as I would call it rape) which resulted in another pregnancy. She was spirited away to a home for unwed mothers where she gave birth to a daughter that she would not meet until she was 87 years old. Fast forward six more years, at 31 years old, after an interval that included losing a fiancé to a heart attack, she conceived another child—my brother. She told the father, the man who would also become my father, she would give birth to and keep the baby with or without him. He is quoted as saying, "He would give having a family a try." That was about as affectionate as things got between the two.

I have yet to mention that my mother was an active alcoholic throughout this. She jokes that if drugs were as accessible as they are now, she would probably be dead. My mom credits my father for saving her life. After two years of marriage, when my brother was twelve months old, he said to her, "I can live with just about anything but a drunk. You either stop drinking or I am leaving." She quit that day and never drank alcohol again. I was conceived at this inflection point. Smoking a pack or two of cigarettes daily, however, would remain her vice for thirteen more years.

"You were afraid of men when you were little," my family would say lightheartedly. They thought it was cute that I would not get on the nursery school bus at age 4 because the driver was a man. As I grew up, I suppressed my trepidation around men, but I clearly remember the relief I felt after getting engaged and having a ring on my finger. It was as if I suddenly had a shield protecting me from potential threats. I have no memory of physical or sexual abuse. Had my father laid his hands on me before I had language capacity or explicit memory? Or did I come into the world with generational and past life trauma that robbed me of the innocence of a carefree childhood through which I could experience the world as a safe and wondrous place? While I now have a strong intuitive and embodied sense that all the above are true, the impact of it all was lodged deep in my subconscious.

I knew little of my mother's history nor had I explored the implications of being afraid of men when my boss, Stan, suggested my new fiancé and I get premarital counseling before we got married. "What? What did we need counseling for?" I thought to myself, rather annoyed this was the way he greeted the news of my engagement. I had snagged a great catch and was headed into the mythical happily ever after so why would I mess with that?

Not only was my soon-to-be husband great looking and wicked smart, but his family also had significant financial means—a near perfect combination when one is intent on being a dependent, kept woman. That intention was so strong that I would overlook a couple obvious red flags. I convinced myself that it would all magically resolve once we were married and committed to one another.

Alongside the defensiveness I felt when my boss posed the premarital counseling option, a faint internal voice made its way into my conscious awareness, and I more thoughtfully considered his invitation. In addition to my fear that if we didn't address immediate issues, I would lose my American Dream relationship, I was also aware that the main models for relationship and marriage were our parents. Wrought with divorce and addictions on both sides, it seemed a potentially good idea to get some support.

I wrote a letter (in today's world it would have been an email or text) to Rich, my fiancé, suggesting we follow my boss's advice and have a session with a couple's therapist for premarital counseling. My reluctance to have a face-to-face conversation reflects the first of many times I would tamp down my desires and limit my full voice.

Rich said he would give the counseling a try. Even with all

the unconscious material surrounding this moment, we made a choice that was way outside both of our comfort zones, unprecedented in either of our families. At 23 years old in 1989, I had no peers going down this path. However reluctantly Rich was to do it, I am so grateful he said yes. This choice would alter the trajectory of our lives.

In one of our early sessions, our therapist asked if my husband and I wanted children. We both said, "Yes! But not right away." He was happy to hear this and advised us to consider dedicating at least a few years to work on ourselves and build a strong foundation for our marriage before taking that step. He proposed that our wedding didn't make us married, it was the kick-off celebration to start being married. This was sound advice we took to heart, and it was reasonable given we were in our mid-twenties.

And work we did! We went deep into our personal work. I soon realized that the American Dream life I had always envisioned for myself was empty and superficial. I had earned a BBA (neither of my parents graduated from college) and was working as an economic analyst with a University of Chicago-trained economist in litigation consulting. Yet, I was awakening to the truth that it was all a back-up plan until the day I could quit, have babies, and hang out at the country club. It was only after acknowledging these shadow truths and building a core sense of myself that I could begin to envision a path that wasn't dictated by my mother's opinions. It was from this space, four years after getting married, that I decided I wanted to go off the birth control pill so I could get my body ready for conceiving, which we both felt was coming soon.

It is often at inflection points such as a marriage, or conception, or divorce that we seek support. I did not realize it at the time, but my choice to engage in premarital counseling was my first act of rewriting the Mother Code. For me it was like the movie *Brave*, where the main character, Merida, is a rebellious princess who rejects the tradition of arranged marriage that her mother, Queen Elinor, tries to impose on her. Merida first believes that escaping tradition is the only way to find freedom. However, she discovers that true liberation lies not in running away from expectations but in reshaping them in ways that honor both her individuality and her family.

Harvesting your childhood codes is an essential part of this process. It is not for the faint of heart, but I also want you to consider how much you are offering to those you love. Yes, we all want what makes us comfortable; of course we do. But the greatest love offerings of all are those that move us beyond comfortable complacence into full-blown actualization. You are offering a gift. The truth of your experience is a treasure to yourself and to those around you. As the sources of your personal Mother Code become apparent to you, and as you move away from the old relationships you had with them, never forget that there is no scarcity in this situation. What is on offer is nothing less than universal, cosmic abundance.

Your Cultural Code

At the heart of the Mother Code is the seemingly endless flow of questions that arise from the moment one thinks about becoming a mother. Because this is an all-encompassing period in the lives of mothers and children, we are all affected by the ideas and actions organized around mothering. The Mother Code is far more than a set of rules about what to do when you are pregnant and raising a child. This scaffolding appears around every creative act, every important life goal, every act of nurturing—the mother and child relationship pervades all of society.

When it seems as though there is evidence of the Mother Code everywhere you look: It *is* everywhere! And it touches everyone no matter where you are on the mothering continuum. If you are raising children, you are bombarded with messages about how to do it that strategically reinforce the paradigm of "intensive mothering."[2] Few women who have raised children in the U.S. in the past few decades have avoided the incessant "do it all" messaging of which intensive mothering is just one of the most troublesome. As awareness of the Mother Code grows, the awareness of the mechanics behind the messaging can be as omnipresent as the messages, showing the whole picture.

This can feel a little claustrophobic at first. It's important to put the Mother Code in perspective. Our understanding of the world largely depends on a mesh of systems like the Mother Code created and maintained by society. All day, you receive messages about what it means to be beautiful, to be feminine or rugged, to love our country, to have faith, to be responsible, and so on. Admittedly, it's a little creepy to realize that so much of what we think of as news, sports, entertainment, and shopping is reinforcement of society's norms, but that is how our brains interact with the world—until we take charge of our own minds. Think of this process as removing a filter to your view of the world so you can better see what is there.

The specific codes targeting mothers are often contradictory and so this filter will be a practical aid and a critical tool in your quest for personal development. Consider, for example, the conflicting pressures to devote every waking moment to children. So many of us feel we are not the women we are supposed to be because we can't do all of this at once, but we are not meant to! You are only one person, and you must make choices about how to divide your precious time.

Before you saw the Mother Code all around you, this may have manifested as a vague sense of guilt, reinforcing earlier anxieties

---

2 Intensive mothering ideology, as described by Hays (1996), consists of a set of beliefs about children and maternal behaviors. Hays organized these beliefs into three domains of focus: (a) sacred children/sacred mothering, (b) the responsibility of individual mothers, and (c) intensive methods of childrearing. Hays, Sharon. *The Cultural Contradictions of Motherhood*. Yale University Press, 1996. For a robust re-evaluation of the concept, see Ennis, Linda Rose. *Intensive Mothering: The Cultural Contradictions of Modern Motherhood*. Demeter Press, 2014.

about whether you were good enough as a mother, as a woman, as a human. We now see behind the veil and know these are constructs without our best interests at heart. It may be uncomfortable at first to recognize how dysfunctional our social cues are, but it is also freeing once you realize that we can reject the irrationality of the system advancing a role for us.

Your *Cosmic Code*

Sometimes, the walls to a garden are so high you cannot see over them. You know something wonderful lies on the other side—you can't see it, but you can feel it!

You: "What is this darn wall doing here? Where did it come from? Why is it here?"

Voice of the Cosmos: "You built the wall."

You: "Wait, what? You are saying *I* built this wall? No way!"

Voice of the Cosmos: "Yes, with the help of your family and the prevailing culture—you all contributed. And as a matter of fact, you marveled at it and praised its height and the sturdiness and thickness of the walls. Everyone around you was doing it and when they added anything to the wall, like paint or more height, you felt compelled to do the same. It is quite an accomplishment!"

You: "I did? No way! Well, I am sure I had my reasons as a child, but I think I may be missing out by not having access to what is inside those walls."

Voice of the Cosmos: "That is true! You were very clever as a little one and those walls served you. The higher and thicker the wall, the more protection you had to survive your situation. It served an important purpose, but you may discover that you do not need it anymore… You can start by putting a window in, then a door, and then eventually you may realize that you are safe and secure without it."

You: "What exactly is on the other side? I feel drawn to it, but also apprehensive."

Voice of the Cosmos: "That is yours to discover! I know the beauty, wisdom, and nourishment that lives on the other side is within your grasp. The important thing is you are on the journey!"

The Cosmic Codes are one of three layers of codes that are part of the Mother Code. The others, Childhood and Cultural Codes, are where the status quo, misconceptions, and limitations of our society's Mother Code are planted. The Cosmic Codes are the source of the true nature of mothering and point the way to growth and transcendence.

I will talk a lot about the other two codes in concrete terms because they are how the code manifests, but the Cosmic Code is always a part of the whole picture, even if it is not always as obvious. When you break down the childhood and cultural walls that sit between you and your enlightened, empowered, and engaged experience of mothering, you open yourself to an experience that is beyond your imagining. I say it is beyond your imagining, not because you are not capable of reaching it. Rather it is because you are standing on the shoulders of generations of women forbidden to consider it, let alone have their needs and desires met.

Part of the experience will be giving yourself permission to dream, to see possibilities and not shut them down immediately. Your families and wider culture are constantly telling you how to mother because it reinforces the walls they built. And until they are ready to topple the edifice themselves, they may not be immediately supportive of your desire to do so. That's okay! Just don't let it stop you from following your urge to merge with the universe and experience the power and sacredness of the Cosmic Codes.

Breaking the Myths of the Mother Code

The limitations surrounding mothering are so insidious in our culture, most of us don't even realize the danger or how we are being undermined at every turn. We are fish swimming in a sea of debris, mistaking it for nourishment. That about 4,530,000,000 (yes 4 billion!) results pop up on a Google search for "how to mother" may seem to be helpful, but it is sending the message that you don't know what the heck you are doing, and worse, that there is apparently a right way to mother. If this was the truth, we would need only one book because it would have all the answers.

In pursuit of an impossible ideal, you are tasked to sift through the mounds of material accessible to you, and if you are anything like me, the more I dive deep into a dizzying number of options and data, the more anxious I feel. That's not to say that some of what is being offered isn't useful. But I hope that this book helps you navigate the tricky seas and distinguish between the harmful debris and genuine nourishment so you can experience the beauty and wonder of the experience.

Myth #1: Pregnancy is a Problem

It is reasonable for us to ask why the pregnancy book called the Bible and a perennial presence on the New York Times bestseller list is all about the worst things that might happen to pregnant women. And the answer tells us a great deal about the Mother Code and how it gets transmitted. While this is a book for mothers in a literal sense, it is also a book for men in a more subtle sense at the same time.

We delayed announcing my first pregnancy so we could have time and space to be with the magic of the experience in our own little bubble. I knew that as soon as I started sharing I was expecting, most of the reaction I would hear would be about how awful it is to be pregnant. I don't think most people intentionally go around trying to discourage pregnant women, but it becomes something of a downer when one comment after the next is about some pregnancy problem.

The first question many people asked me—and ask all pregnant women—is when I was due. Because I had an August due date, I was inundated with comments about how hot and uncomfortable I would be and to prepare to suffer through the whole third trimester because it was in the summer. All of it was intended to signal sympathy, of course, but it still sounds a lot like you're just telling everyone some bad news.

"Oh, that's gonna be so *awful*."

"You'll be *miserable* all summer."

This kind of sympathy, I could have done without.

And then there was all the advice which amounted to more predictions of how terrible the experience would be. I was told my back would hurt, that I would end up waddling, and all sorts of other problems women had experienced. Nobody was trying to be negative, but the problems of pregnancy were the main focus of a whole lot of the conversations I had about my status as a newly pregnant mom.

And you know what, a lot of this is repeating what we've been told or our own experience as if it is the same for everyone. When I was told waddling was inevitable, I was curious, and I questioned the validity of that statement. Sure enough, I hit a point in pregnancy where I waddled. I didn't want to waddle, so instead of taking it as fact, I figured out how to adjust my stride given my new proportions.

Some women talked about their bodies as if all strength had been sapped from them, but I decided to continue to exercise during both of my pregnancies. My trainer mentioned more than once that my strength and stamina had *increased*. They said, "You should be pregnant all the time!" I eased back into my exercise routine postbirth, and it felt great. Yet I also recall one friend specifically telling me she read women should limit and even curtail exercise as if it were a medical fact. (And it wouldn't surprise me if it is presented that way to women.)

I was not any more physically prepared for my pregnancy than a lot of other women are, but I was skeptical about the idea that I would become helpless for months on end because I was going to have a baby. I challenged assumptions, and I learned a lot of those truisms are made from a one-size-fits-all perspective and do not consider what works on a person-by-person basis. In a small but significant way, I was already seeing the outlines of a Mother Code that did not allow me agency but instead instructed me to adopt an attitude of unknowing helplessness.

Myth #2: Birth is a Medical Event

Birth is unequivocally an event—at once mundane as well as won-drous—that perpetuates humanity. It has the power to reveal the mysteries of creation and cycles of life with the woman as a sacred vessel in partnership with the child she has been carrying and brings into the world through the portal of her body. For eons, birth was held in the highest regard and a symbol of a woman's power and manifested in physical form. Birth as a medical event, conversely, is a Western, masculinized cultural construct with a beginning marked by the gleaming sign as she drives up to the hospital—EMERGENCY.[3]

Pretty much immediately upon entry, a monitoring device is attached to the lower belly, which is itself a shocking experience given the sensitivity of that area, and there is no longer a need to consult the delivering mother regarding essential aspects of the experience such as heart rate and contractions. If the monitor does not register a big contraction, it's not a big contraction even if mom says it is; the monitor now churns out data that takes precedence.

This is important enough to repeat: Birth is not a medical emer-gency, until it is. There is no advantage and a number of disadvan-tages to behave otherwise. The Mother Code tells us we should be terrified, rather than stepping into one of the most monumental experiences of our life conscious and prepared.

---

3   Here are two excellent sources if you are interested in a deeper discussion of the medical-ization of birth—and I will be providing more in future chapters: Odent, Michel. "The Masculinisation of the Birth Environment." *Journal of Prenatal and Perinatal Psychology and Health* 23.3 (2009); Downe, Susan, ed. *Normal Childbirth: Evidence and Debate.* Elsevier Health Sciences, 2008.

Birth centers take the opposite approach—as do home births, by their very nature. In both instances, the operating premise is that birth is natural and ordinary—*because it is*. The first thing that made this approach attractive was primal. It was all about the food for me. Most births in a hospital include food deprivation, largely to prepare for the possible need for a cesarean section. When I heard that having a home birth meant I could eat what I want when I want, it won me over right away.

Lighting is another underappreciated difference between the two experiences. Hospital lights are perhaps the most intrusive, unpleasant form of lighting. Birthing centers are lit like homes, and that can play a significant part in reducing the stress and anxiety of a birth. In a crisis-oriented approach to birth, things like food and lighting seem trivial, when in reality a birthing woman's sensitivity to space and having basic needs met are foundational for her to surrender to the waves of the experience.

And let's talk about losing the sacredness of the event. It would seem natural that an experience that began in the privacy of your bedroom, where you have the freedom to cry out through the razor's edge line between pain and pleasure and exclaim, "Oh God!" should culminate in that same space. Can you imagine the sweaty, messy, explosive act of making a baby taking place at Gate 5 of the airport with all the crew changeovers, and people milling about? That is what we ask of women giving birth in many hospital settings.

I am grateful for the medical technology that has brought effective life-saving measures when needed. But sadly, this system has created a powerful hierarchy of dependence. Having lost sight of the original intention to heal, it has become a bureaucratic institution that is more concerned with accumulating impersonal transactions.

We need to upend this disempowering terminology of birth as a medical event and return it to a space where a woman connects with her divine wisdom encoded in her body that is *supported* by scientific knowledge, not run by it. And when I say "return to a space," I mean that quite literally. I urge everyone reading this book to become knowledgeable about midwives, doulas, birthing centers, and home birth. You are the architect of your birthing experience. This is one of the greatest losses of power caused by the medicalization of birthing.

You have a choice, and centering yourself in your birth should be a high priority for you and those who will take part in the birth.

Myth #3: Modern Parenting Is an Ancient Rite

My mom would always say that her 40s were her favorite decade because that's when she had us. For my mom, parenting was something you did to get your needs met. My parents did not have a romantic relationship. It was plainly transactional, with my father providing for the family materially and largely wanting to be left alone when he got home. My brother and I were where my mother came for love and affection and to feel needed.

In many ways, this is the model that we have been told is the blueprint; it is simply the way families have existed for time immemorial. We have arrived at our current understanding of the idea of motherhood through a journey that can be traced from the 1800s to the present. I often call the current era's approach the medicalization of motherhood and birth. Others have used "scientific motherhood."[4] The longer this period goes on, the more the women it caters to come to expect medical support for some or all aspects of conception, pregnancy, and birth—and even to depend on it (psychologically if not physiologically). The net effect of this dependency is to blot out the insight that mothers have the power to lead and guide pregnancy and birth and should be followed and not led.

---

4 Rima Apple's excellent book, *Perfect Motherhood*, traces the history and development of this period of "scientific motherhood" and is an engaging read. Full citation: Apple, Rima. *Perfect Motherhood: Science and Childrearing in America.* New Brunswick, NJ: Rutgers University Press, 2006.

I contrast my parents' relationship with that of my grandparents—both their relationship to each other and to us. My grandmother never had to seek the affection she might have wanted from her husband. He showed his love for her every day—and she reciprocated. They were both loving toward me too, and every summer, they would live with us. That's where I saw a couple having sweet exchanges and enjoying each other's company. This is not part of the two-parents, 2.5-kids blueprint we are told is the correct way to raise children. But if it wasn't for this nonconformist family structure, I would have lost what was probably the most important model for a loving relationship I saw during my formative years.

Myth #4: There Is One Way to Mother

A debilitating and harmful myth that sprouts in our families and takes root in our culture is that there is a one (right) way to mother. Generally, it starts with well-meaning family members showing you *how it is done* and innocently passing the baton. In my case, if I asked my mother for advice and I didn't follow it, she would get angry and say, "If you aren't going to follow my advice then don't ask my opinion." We laugh about it now, but oh my, the audacity in this statement! I am not alone when I say the result of growing up with domineering mothers or family members is that you begin to doubt yourself—at least I did.

That wiring was deeply worn into my neurocircuitry. When listening to people like doctors or coaches who had high opinions of themselves and felt their word was truth beyond reproach, I was quick to jump on board. Why should I waste my energy thinking or having an opinion when they clearly know their stuff?

Rewriting the Parenting Paradigm

It may come as a surprise, but the term "parenting," so ubiquitous in our current culture, has not always existed. Before industrialization, children were expected to contribute to the family starting at an early age. They had responsibilities to help maintain the family business—be it a kingdom or a farm. But when the income-producing labor for the family began to shift to the sole responsibility of the parents and happened outside the home, the system was upended. Instead of the child being of service to the family, the parents were of service to the child.

Dr. Alison Gopnik, professor of psychology at UC Berkeley, shares about this in her book, *The Gardener and the Carpenter: What the New Science of Child Development Tells Us About the Relationship Between Parents and Children*, when she made the distinction between parenting as a job and "being a parent." The job of parenting was an innovation that got started in the 1950s and took hold in the 1970s and became a process much like school (which is modeled after a factory assembly line) and employment where you are expected to produce something and then be graded, evaluated, and linearly promoted based on your output.

Gopnik's framework uses the metaphor of a carpenter, where you use specific tools to chisel and mold your child into the successful adult that fits your picture and that of the current culture's ideal. It is neat, orderly, and predictable. Good luck with that! Raising a child is anything but predictable! And our continuous attempts to regulate it is like trying to control the weather. No wonder we experience so much frustration and angst as parents. No wonder children feel stifled under our over-worrying and over-doing for them.

Being a gardener offers a more nuanced, and messy, experience. When you plant a garden, you become a steward of the land and the growth that emerges from it. You will provide nourishment and protection for the seeds you plant so they can grow and thrive and become themselves. A garden requires getting dirty, it is a messy and chaotic endeavor, but you weather the storms and watch in wonder as the natural alchemy of the elements grows a tiny seed into a beautiful plant or tree or flower. You may have known what the seed would turn into, but you appreciate its unique beauty. The gardener is not worried if the seed they planted turned out right, they appreciate it as it is.

Children flourish when given freedom. This doesn't mean no boundaries or guiderails are put into place. But studies show that when children are in large open spaces with no fence they stay in one small area, but when a boundary is marked with a fence or tree line, they explore the whole space. The size of this space expands and grows with them.

I am further struck with the question Gopnik asks at the start of the book: "Why be a parent?"[5] She cites research that reflects how our noble intentions and everything we do for our children doesn't correlate to particular outcomes. If it is not a verb or form of work or sculpting a child into a particular adult, what is it? Gopnik puts it this way: "Instead, to be a parent—to care for a child—is to be part of a profound and unique human relationship, to engage in a particular kind of love."[6] This recentering of how we mother is in powerful relationship to Rewriting the Mother Code.

Isn't it loving to want your child to go to Harvard or become a CEO of a company? Sure, you want your children to be safe and to thrive, but it's good to be curious about your own projections. The question to ask here is, whose dream is it to graduate from an Ivy League school? Maybe you dreamed of becoming an actor on Broadway, but your parents communicated loud and clear that the performing arts could be a hobby but not a career.

Now guess what happens when you have a child of your own? You put them in theatre camp and any way of performing arts schools and classes not even noticing how much they love playing with puzzles and could do math problems all day long. Our children

---

5 Gopnik, Alison. *The Gardener and the Carpenter: What the New Science of Child Development Tells Us About the Relationship Between Parents and Children.* Macmillan, 2016, 3.

6 Gopnik, 9.

are not our vehicle to live vicariously through. But we can learn about ourselves as we venture to see our children fully as themselves. I had always wanted to learn to play an instrument. I begged my parents to get a drum set, but I would have settled for any instrument. My parents said it would be too loud and that I would get bored with it after a short time, so the answer was, "No!" The answer was no for similar reasons to tap dancing and getting a sewing machine. Imagine what was wired in my belief system about valuing my creativity, making noise, and seeing things through to the end. Well, if I couldn't do those things I wanted in my childhood, my children were going to.

So, guess who got her children started on Suzuki violin at age 3—me! I had all the data to support how valuable it was to start a child young on an instrument and that the violin, while difficult, was the best one to develop a good ear for music. It was frustrating and I ignored their dislike of the whole endeavor until I was in a life coaching session that revealed *I* wanted to play an instrument. It was an unhealed childhood wound.

Guess who started her own violin lessons—me! Soon, we were all learning together. I was able to be more empathetic as I experienced first-hand how difficult the instrument was, but also the joy of sticking with it and learning a song. To have the teacher tell me I was naturally good at it was both music to my ears and bittersweet. I was hurt and angry about the missed opportunity in my own youth, and I was rewiring old beliefs around giving myself space for creative expression, making mistakes as a pathway to learning was not a reason to quit, and most importantly the experience of not living *through* my children, but living *with* them.

This possibility for mothers and fathers to learn and grow with our children is something I want to keep top of mind. To love ourselves and then share that love with our children is the framework we are exploring on these pages. We all have baggage and unhealed wounds from our childhoods that get in the way of loving ourselves. Rather than foisting the fears, hurts, and resentments buried in our unconscious onto our children, we can recognize them and learn how they may be reactively influencing our parenting choices. Once they are out in the open, we have the sacred opportunity for self-compassion and healing.

There is more dysfunction in the parenting paradigm we will not be getting into, such as the disparity of how billions are spent on parenting books, yet we have children and teens experiencing more depression and anxiety than ever before. Despite our obsession with test scores, our literacy rates are low and getting lower, especially in lower-income households. Parents are under tremendous stress and exhausted from the labor of raising children. These are all important issues surrounding parenting. While I am not addressing them directly, I hope that by debunking myths and providing a process that opens us to more responsible decision making around child-rearing, we can create a culture that brings to bear the strengths of mothers and fathers harmonizing feminine and masculine principles.

Rewriting the Motherhood Paradigm

I hope it is becoming abundantly clear that motherhood is a cultural construct. We are fish in water, and we flow with the currents of our society's prevailing notions of what it means to mother. It is our responsibility to come up for air, look around, and see the landscape with eyes wide open and with a willingness to explode commonly held beliefs and behaviors that are familiar, but not always in our best interest as mothers.

The current atmosphere for mothering is crumbling under the weight of unrealistic expectations and underappreciated contributions. We are failing as a society to provide an experience that lets a woman thrive and shine in her full power and infuse mother energy into all her spheres. More women are opening up about the challenges they face in our current culture. We have at least

6,000 years of patriarchal domination to unravel, and while we are making progress because of many brave women speaking up and challenging the status quo, we need to accelerate the pace. I trust in humanity's ability to acknowledge where we are wrong and steer the ship through and out of the fog. We have done it before, but we have also ignored the fog horns and met our doom. Join me in sounding the call and making our voices heard.

We have all resources to shift the prevailing winds away from a dysfunctional system to a structure that centers mothers' experience first on their own care and nourishment and then on their children. Andrea O'Reilly, author, professor, founder of Motherhood Studies (2006), and creator of the concept of Matricentric Feminism, makes it clear that we must insist on the value of development during the mothering process as a benefit to mothers as human beings, not simply to the extent it makes us better parents. Rewriting the Mother Code inherently achieves this imperative, as the distinction between raising a child and nourishing a mother combines into one dynamic unity of purpose.

As O'Reilly notes in her important anthology *Mother Outlaws*, children—and especially daughters—literally cannot see their mothers as complete human beings when she is "perceived and understood only in terms of her maternal identity."[7] Even when one considers the value of the development of a mother to her children, remaining subjugated under a masculine-defined set of rules fails the whole family in terms of achieving personal growth. "[W]e must eradicate oppressive motherhood," O'Reilly declares, "and achieve emancipatory mothering *for mothers themselves*, so that they may be enriched and empowered by mothering."[8]

---

7 O' Reilly, Andrea, ed. *Mother Outlaws: Theories and Practices of Empowered Mothering.* Canadian Scholars and Women's Press, 2004, 61.

8 O' Reilly, 72.

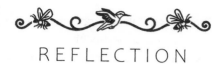

REFLECTION

Return to conscious awareness of your breath and use these questions to reflect on your experience:

What did you notice about your breathing as you engaged with this chapter?

Did something you read make you gasp?

Were you holding your breath at any point?

Did you breathe a sigh of recognition as some myths of motherhood were shared out loud?

Bringing increased awareness to your breath will give you opportunities to regulate your emotions and embrace all that comes your way on your mothering expedition.

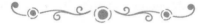

More and more, I realize that transformation never ends, and I am continually learning and growing—particularly when I look through the lens of my mothering. I recently had the blessing of coaching a woman through her mothering choices surrounding conception, pregnancy, and birth. Just as emotions and triggers arise to be honored and healed while directly mothering a child, they also come up when coaching someone else in that process.

After spending time with Liza and her newborn in their home, I was gripped with sadness. Her capacity to be present with herself and then with her newborn was palpable. It was beautiful to witness, but highlighted ways the overwhelm, fears, and doubts accompanying new motherhood had consumed me. As I seemed to uncover a new layer of the onion of my self-awareness, I brought this realization into my own coaching and was reminded this was not something I needed to feel guilty about.

This was an opportunity for radical compassion around my mothering. My coach asked me to consider what I needed that didn't come directly from me. I realized I had needed massive comfort and encouragement by my husband and a "mom"—the same amount or more that I received during the birth I needed in spades as a new mother. There was not enough care, and it was not my fault. It was liberating to take that weight off my heart and put the onus on the systemic problems that led to me not receiving the care I needed.

How beautiful the experience of learning and growing as a mother is. I met an Irish author, Morgan Llwelyn, and she said that when someone asks how she is doing instead of saying "fine" she says, "I am grappling with the immensities." What a blessing it is to be alive! It's a gift to have the opportunity to grapple with my own immensities and know that the energy of such endeavors will ripple outward, potentially affecting my family and women across the globe.

We are all in the dance of the immensities.

Chapter 3

Expressing Your Motherhood

When I did not get pregnant a few months into having sex to conceive, I started to get nervous. I began to realize there was so much I didn't know about the whole conception process itself,[1] let alone my own body and its cycles. This would become the first stop in my quest for conception.

When we first started out intentionally conceiving, I was all about creating a sacred space. I would light candles and make sure everything was inviting and welcoming. As months went by, it became more and more difficult to hold any sacred space or specialness around our lovemaking. It became a task. There were plenty of times we were impersonal and robotic because we were

---

1 A common challenge, though not everyone realizes how much she doesn't know: Lundsberg, Lisbet S., et al. "Knowledge, attitudes, and practices regarding conception and fertility: a population-based survey among reproductive-age United States women." *Fertility and Sterility* 101.3 (2014): 767-774. https://www.sciencedirect.com/science/article/pii/S0015028213034250.

within the brief window of ovulation. I wanted to be one of those women I read stories about who knew and felt the moment of conception in profound ways. But after a while I didn't give a rat's ass about that. I just wanted to get pregnant. Wrestling with all the uncertainty of when or even if I would conceive was starting to weigh on me. I remained hopeful but was wondering if or when we would need a fertility specialist. My struggles were not a failure but a testament to the complex interplay of biological factors and societal expectations.

It was right around this time that my husband and I set out on our annual pilgrimage to sacred sites around the world—a time of year where we stepped out of the temporal routine of our lives and focused on nourishing our spirit in a remembering and reawakening of the mystical side of life. Along with 25 men and women from diverse backgrounds and religious and spiritual orientations, we set out to explore the country of Ireland. My husband and I shared with the group that we were trying to conceive and would love support and energy and encouragement while we were in these sacred spaces.

This admission was vulnerable and was breaking rules about conception being a private matter, one that Rich and I should handle on our own. It was touching to have the support of the group and we felt honored to be included. One woman gave us a little totem that represented fertility to her. At one of the many ancient stone circle sites we visited throughout the trip, the group bestowed visions and blessings on us, and we ended it with a light-hearted made-up ritual.

This was all sweet and lovely, and I practiced receiving so much love and attention. But it was at an unplanned stop along one of our driving days I had a profound mystical experience. Our coach driver suggested we make a stop at a roadside grotto dedicated to Mother Mary. Mind you, these are abundant in the predominantly

Catholic country of the Republic of Ireland, but he had personal experience with one he wanted to share with us.

We got out off the bus and right there on the roadside was a small open area. Off to the right a short distance away were stone steps that led to a little alcove where a gleaming white statue of Mary stood. There were offerings of flowers all around her and candles lit holding wishes and prayers of others who came to Her. We were guided to meditate silently as we took in the space. I kneeled in front of the Mary statue and prayed my usual prayer asking for support with my desire to conceive. We were getting ready to head back to the bus when one of the participants spontaneously started singing Ave Maria. Her voice sounded even more beautiful than usual, and I closed my eyes and let the angelic sounds wash over me. It was in this moment of opening I heard a voice say...

"You and Rich are a family, whether you have a child or not."

These words pierced my heart, and I sobbed as I let this simple but astonishingly profound truth reverberate through my whole being. Within the container of this spiritual transmission, the cloak of illusion that conceiving a child was my only path to a life of meaning and fulfillment was lifted off my shoulders.

I shared my experience with Rich and then the group. With each retelling, I felt the deepening of an invitation to expand my limiting definitions of family and mothering. I returned home with a profound sense I had experienced a deep healing and an initiation in the mysteries of life.

We conceived the following month.

Was it a miracle? Was it a coincidence? I feel uncomfortable claiming a miracle, but I do not brush off experiences that feel beyond my cognitive reality. I get chills and teary to this day when I share this encounter and that is enough *data* for me to honor it with reverence and gratitude.

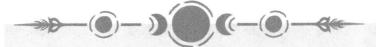

SOUND RITUAL

Voices and sounds from others can serve as a mystical portal like they were for me in the experience I shared above. They can also shut us down and divert us from carving our own unique path. The more we tune into our own voice, the more we can attune with voices that resonate with our highest intentions.

Place your hands gently on your throat, feeling the warmth of your touch and the steady rhythm of your breath. Visualize a soft, warm light glowing at your throat, radiating outward with each breath you take. This light represents the essence of your voice—your unique sound, your truth, your ability to communicate and express yourself. Feel this light expanding with each inhale, growing brighter and more vibrant.

As you continue to breathe, begin to hum softly. Let the hum resonate from deep within, feeling the vibration in your throat and chest. Let the hum be gentle, without force, simply letting your voice emerge naturally. With each hum, imagine the light in your throat becoming more radiant, filling your entire body with warmth and energy. Imagine it connecting with the world around you, sending out waves of your unique energy, your truth. After a few moments, let the hum fade naturally, and return to silence.

Place your hands back on your throat, feeling the energy that still lingers. Whisper softly to yourself: "My voice is powerful, my voice is beautiful, my voice is my truth."

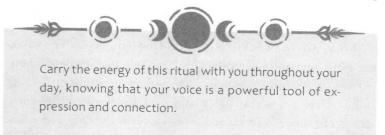

Carry the energy of this ritual with you throughout your day, knowing that your voice is a powerful tool of expression and connection.

Find Your Voice

My story is not a formula, and it is just one of many possibilities—authentic, vulnerable, and relatable. It's a true tale that exposes the beauty woven into the uncertainties; the triumphs nestled within the vulnerabilities. It's a beacon lighting the way for you to navigate your unique path, armed with the wisdom of the ages and the courage to redefine motherhood on your terms.

I am grateful that this part of our story resulted in a pregnancy, and I am aware that it might not have worked out that way. I am also aware that when I engaged in using my voice to rewrite my Mother Codes, I transformed. My thinking expanded. Cells in my body were rearranged. A change occurred that offered me more tools, more wisdom, and more resilience to move forward on my journey.

Like a novitiate taking the first steps toward a deepened faith, the beginning of this process will require regular reminders of what you are seeing and remaking in your life. One way to think about how the building blocks of transformation are interrelated is to consider overarching elements together in a single conceptual framework. VOICE is this framework.

Distilled to its essence, *VOICE* can be summarized this way:

Vision—Mother energy fuels my deepest desires.
Ownership—I unapologetically claim my space.
Intuition—My heart shines a guiding radiant light.
Culture—I create a community of loving support.
Engage—I walk with true steps toward my vision.

I had barely an inkling of what I would encounter as I entered this new world of motherhood. I sensed that it would require self-awareness, but I was only a handful of years into my growth and development where, like a baby bird discovering it has wings and can fly, I was both excited about this new freedom and erratic and wobbly. I had spent my life up to that point looking outside of myself for validation. This was rooted in my enmeshed relationship with my mother. Until shortly after getting engaged and starting growth work, I did not make a move in my life without approval from her or someone I considered an authority. I had the chameleon-like ability of fitting into my surroundings and adopting whatever voice was the authority around me. To build a core sense of self and find my voice, I needed a vision.

While I did not have the VOICE framework to work with explicitly throughout my years of mothering children, my core sense of self was formed from the stories I have shared and more you will hear in the coming pages. I have experienced first-hand over the years that without a *vision* to orient to, we are susceptible to falling into our preprogrammed wiring—some of which is helpful and some that is less than ideal. For me, orienting to consciousness, an embodied, present, and engaged human experience of life as a vision, was a guiding light. It lit my way as I navigated through the many options for conception, pregnancy, birth, and new motherhood. Later you will hear more about where I turned my back on my vision in new motherhood and regressed to old wiring because it felt safe.

Living in a time where women have more agency over their bodies, but not completely (in truth it is limited), I found it critical to take *ownership* of the conception and birth process to have an experience that resonated with me. Had I not known about alternative ways to deal with conception issues, I would have assumed that what my OBGYN told me was the best and only way. In our culture, it is harder to distinguish between manipulation and true care. The lines are blurred between systems that care more about profit and control than they do healthy, happy, empowered birthing outcomes for mothers and babies. If you don't know you have choices in how you want to birth your baby and raise your child, you are essentially being held captive.

I am so grateful for the times I followed my *intuition,* and so remorseful about the times I did not. I worked hard to move away from a culture that dictates how I should feel and how I am supposed to act, but sometimes the wiring is so strong it is difficult to decipher. We overvalue the Yang ideals of timelines, logic, and scientific proof for everything that we engage in. Don't get me wrong, I love research. I love we can prove validity and test outcomes with data and science. But I like to engage with it from the perspective of *backing up* what I already know or feel inside. When we were deciding between a hospital or home birth, I was happy to discover that positive birth outcomes were significantly higher in home births. This was research shared by my home birth midwives as hospitals rarely feel obliged to share this data or show the differences in approaches so we can make informed choices.

Our current Western—and particularly U.S.—culture surrounding motherhood is clogged with misinformation and taboos, reliance on technology and medicalization, and overconsumption of material goods. But the most challenging aspect of our current culture is the isolation women encounter in new motherhood. We no longer live in tribes or large family units. People who do not have family or a close chosen tribe only get support and help when they pay for it. This is less of an issue for privileged and affluent mothers, but devasting for low-income, marginalized communities. New motherhood is hard! For me, creating a culture of community and not being alone in my mothering was challenging— even with the resources I had available.

In addition to the lack of a support system, my covert competitiveness with other mothers coupled with my insecurity kept me further isolated. At the same time, I also experienced the possibility to both live independently and in community with like-minded and caring people. When a tribe is not automatically built in and ready-made, with intention and discernment, the opportunity to choose and create our tribe with people aligned with our values is extraordinary and empowering.

Engaging in life as a conscious human being is nothing short of awesome! I treasure the flashes where I have felt in the present moment with myself, my husband, and my children. Whether these moments were hard-earned through personal growth work or gifts from the universe that I noticed, they are priceless.

It is challenging to put into words, but presence is about those times where you are so in the flow and connected with yourself and those around you that everything else falls away. After one of our daughter's soccer games, rather than dash off quickly to the next thing on our packed weekend agenda, we chose to hang around the field and kick the ball around as a family. We relaxed into play, it wasn't competitive, it wasn't a lesson in soccer, it was fun, and it was freedom. When we chose to spontaneously engage in an activity without the usual agendas, I noticed the difference. I let the feelings of this experience of flow and connection touch me deeply, in a way that let me appreciate it and be nourished by it. We can engage in a lot of activities, but it takes a conscious effort and awareness to be present to them and receive the energy as nourishment.

Vision

The true north of this endeavor is a life in which you are growing in personal development and enriching the lives of you and your loved ones through your rewritten Mother Code. It is an achievable goal, and you will always have your vision to refer to whenever the process feels difficult or frustrating.

Life without a vision is like being in a sailboat without a rudder—moving at the whim of nature without a course in mind or ability to navigate the seas we encounter. We may have a course in mind but no means to steer us toward it, so the circumstances around us dictate our way. With a rudder, however, you can chart a course for the voyage YOU want to go on. While we can't predict every storm that lies ahead veering us off our path, the rudder can steer us back in the direction we intended.

Back when we were trying to conceive our first child, I was introduced to the possibility that healing could come in many forms and modalities and not just from someone wearing a white coat and carrying a stethoscope. I formulated a holistic team approach that included kinesiology, nutrition, homeopathy, and acupuncture as well as therapy and breathwork.

Not one to put all my eggs in one basket (no pun intended!), and because I do also respect Western medicine, I also sought the advice of my gynecologist. Dr. Elena Kamel had come highly recommended and although young was already considered a top OBGYN in Chicago's leading hub for medicine—Northwestern Memorial Hospital. When I presented my circumstances, she let me know that I was suffering from amenorrhea (pronounced ey-men-uh-REE-uh). In addition to sounding like gonorrhea, it had an ominous tone and filled me with dread and fear! I later learned that it's simply the medical term for "lack of menstrual period." She shared her recommendation…I would go on a drug that stimulated ovulation which should induce menstruation. Then, if after a couple months, that didn't work, she would give me the card of a fertility doctor.

I also met with a woman who was trained and practiced as a medical doctor initially but unsatisfied with the limitations also incorporated Chinese medicine. This combination felt good as a balance of both Western and Eastern medicine. I was right, but it wasn't her knowledge in either area that impressed me, it was her powers of observation and being with me that unlocked an obvious but overlooked part of my current state.

She asked me, "Has anyone mentioned that you are very thin?" Wow! Of course! Even I knew that low body fat was often a factor in lack of menstruation. She then astutely pointed out that she could tell me to gain weight, but likely there was an emotional part to this that I would need to uncover to let that happen.

My personal growth coaching and therapy at this point was focused mainly on uncovering any emotional blocks manifesting physically. I was seeking answers to questions like, "What purpose might maintaining a teenage body serve for me?" and "What is in the way of me filling out my curves and stepping into my full womanhood?" I was exploring the edges of my being through dynamic breathwork and biofeedback sessions followed by body work sessions. It was during one of these combination biofeedback-breathwork-bodywork sessions I stepped through a door I had yet to open. I was bent over my coach's knee, almost in a backbend, intended to open my heart, and as I breathed into the strain of this uncomfortable posture, I touched a place of deep awareness.

It was the kind of truth I had kept heavily guarded and tucked away deep in my unconsciousness until I was ready to encounter it. When this truth came through it was not gentle, it hit me like a rocket...

I was terrified to be a mother!

Tears came pouring out. I kept going, breathing into the pain, breathing into the fear. A few moments later the second rocket landed. I was struck again with an even more explosive truth. I wasn't just scared to be mother outright...

I was scared to be a mother like my mother had been...and I didn't want to do that to a child.

I continued to let the tears flow. I welcomed the waves of fear and pain. I invited them to wash over and through me, cleansing and healing as only tears can do. As the tumult eased, an awareness bubbled into my present moment reality...

I was free.

Suddenly it all made sense, my early childhood fear of men, my late start to menstruation (I was 17), staying thin, and keeping a teenage body. My programming dictated that I wanted children, but my body was holding all my past emotional trauma and responded by shutting down the possibility of it happening.

I further realized this wasn't just about my enmeshed, co-dependent relationship with my mother. No, the pain and terror were too deep and old for that. What I experienced was a cathartic release of generational trauma. My mother had her faults—recovering alcoholic, domineering, and controlling to name a few—and I adopted unhealthy coping mechanisms to navigate these challenges in my childhood. But it is now so clear that the level of terror I felt in that moment of the possibility of recreating old patterns went beyond my childhood wounds.

Within a month of this epiphany, everything shifted into place, and I started menstruating. Each new awareness was like finding a piece to a puzzle and the emotional unlocking was the last piece needed to form the whole picture. Some may ask, "So, what is the big deal here? I don't see what the problem is—you ended up menstruating [and eventually as I will share later, conceiving and giving birth to two daughters]. Who cares how you got there?"

Comments like these are often the narrative surrounding pregnancy and birth. The woman's needs, physically and emotionally, are often eclipsed by the goal of conceiving and birthing a baby rather than a woman creating and being guided by a vision that puts herself at the center of this part of her life path.

Why don't more women begin their mothering journey by creating a meaningful vision for themselves? How has it come to be that the first step women automatically take in their conception journey is to take prenatal vitamins? Somehow that message, while not unimportant but sadly limited in scope, has landed. Having a vision helped me discern and question and be curious. It helped me meet the "norm" head on and challenge traditional notions.

What I want you to understand at this juncture is that, inside, you know what you want. You know what you value. You know what your gifts are. You have senses and pictures of the experience you desire. Let those come to the surface. Open yourself to possibilities and dreams. Watch out for any negative or critical thoughts that try to minimize or diminish your ideals as you awaken to them. Understand that is only the wiring from our families and culture that keeps us from stepping into the life we deeply yearn for, and it is why we need a powerful vision to navigate through the fog that would otherwise immobilize us.

Ownership

The Mother Code is a mirror to our lives, reflecting all aspects of our human world, including the messy ones. This is a central reason taking control of it is so important—it influences every part of who you are whether you want it to or not. Mothers can't afford to ignore the uncomfortable parts of life. The kinds of experiences many of us avoid—intense pain, funky messes, sleepless nights—are routine for mothers, from birth, throughout our lives.

Mothers go where others cannot or will not go. This includes the process through which you will rewrite the Mother Code to serve your growth and development and that of your families. And that's why we will talk about *ownership,* a topic we cannot deny is central to the way all of us live. To ignore it is to ignore some of the most powerful assumptions written into the Mother Code.

Who has ultimate control over what we do and how we do it? It is so tempting to adopt a worldview which does not fit us correctly, like an outfit off the rack that is a little long in the legs and narrow in the waist. Your self, your body, and your mind should feel tailor-made. You have a right to feel comfortable and safe in your body and mind. And in this world, that means you have the right to declare ownership over your body.

In an earlier time, the fight for ownership of one's self as a woman was more overt, with women needing to wrestle from society basic rights like voting and property ownership. A couple of years ago, I would have added control over one's body to that list, but as of this writing, we've returned to a place where that is very much in question.

How can I own my body if I fear it? How can I own my body, particularly the parts that physically make me a woman, if my religion, my mother, my father, teachers, and the media are programming me with messages of impurity, shame, inconvenience, and objectivity, to name but a few? However deep and insistent the messaging has been for you will gauge how significant the rewriting of the story of your body will be. We must first know our body to own it. V's international best-selling book, and Tony Award-winning play, *Vagina Monologues* is as relevant today as when it came out in 1996.

Knowing, honoring, valuing, and owning my body has been, and continues to be, a lifelong quest for me. One such meeting of my body came while I was first trying to conceive, and it is one I hold dear. I call this anecdote, "The Sticky Intelligence of Vaginal Mucus." Now if you immediately said or thought, "Eww!" or "Gross!" then be warned, I am unapologetically going into the mysterious and beautiful territory of the vagina!

While only a few months into intentionally trying to conceive, fear was seeping into my consciousness. I was not doing any formal tracking, just having sex and hoping we would hit the mark. "Hmm," I thought, "I better step up my game here." Then I asked a MD friend, who knew the conscious conception journey I was on, to support me. She was respectfully and honored to oblige. So there, in the safety and comfort of my home, my friend guided me through Reproduction 101.

While the basics were familiar I was shocked at how much I

didn't know! My menstrual cycle was always irregular and could vary from four to sometimes eight weeks, which made it tricky to pinpoint when I was ovulating. This was well before Apps and other modern ways to track cycles, so I started a handwritten chart where I monitored my temperature and other bodily sensations every day.

Sidenote here...I have a love-hate relationship with the technology and devices that track our physical cycles because they can also distance us from connection to our actual body. I would suggest using them thoughtfully and with your intuition and body signals, not in place of them.

My forever favorite part of this data-gathering adventure was learning from my friend that one of the most accurate ways to track my cycle was by observing my vaginal mucus! It turns out mucus provides the most valuable information in real time. Here I thought vaginal mucus was just this smelly stuff emitted from my body whose main function was lubrication for sex—was I wrong! By scooping a little on my finger and pressing it between my thumb and forefinger and observing its consistency and stickiness I could tell where I was in my cycle. This was truly a mind-blowing discovery! You mean if I tune in to it, my own body can actually give me the information I need?

If this is new to you too, I strongly urge you to connect with your body in this way. It is so beautifully intimate. Even if conception is not on your radar, tuning into the powerful rhythms of your body and marveling at the wonders of your earthly vessel is worth the effort.

I learned that throughout a woman's cycle the mucus goes from dry (not fertile), to sticky (not fertile), to creamy (semi-fertile), to wet and stretchy, like egg whites (fertility magic). I loved that during the potent time of ovulation the discharge was called *spin*. This term was both delightful and somehow magical sounding but it also made sense because this was the only time the substance held together when I pulled my fingers apart, creating a slippery pathway for sperm to swim to the egg. While I was enthralled with this discovery, it was bittersweet. I realized just how out of touch (literally!) I was from my body and unaware of the natural cycles it goes through every month.

The other beautiful act of support my doctor friend provided me was showing me around everything housed within my pelvic girdle, aka my womb. This hands-on tour included a speculum (there must be a better way!) and a mirror. Yes, it was vulnerable and squirmy, but with someone whom I trusted and felt safe with, it was so empowering. Juxtapose this experience with a typical gyno visit where I bear through the discomfort and wait for the doctor to tell me how my body is functioning—from their perspective.

Let's get the mirrors out, women, and look at our lady parts— inside and out! It is quite wondrous and beautiful. In so doing, you say good riddance to the shame woven into our culture, and sadly trauma, surrounding everything "down there." Venture into territory that most women never think about, let alone take the time to go to, and explore this incredible system.

Most importantly you will affirm the ownership of your physical body!

Own your body. Own your being. No one knows your body better than you. And, if like me, you don't know her—get to know her. Be kind to her and protect her. You decide who you share your body with and when.

Intuition

The Mother Code as it is instilled in us extends far beyond what we think of as *just mothering* and includes a broader hedging in of women in the world, marginalizing our influence and reframing our unique strengths as weaknesses. Without question, intuition has been devalued when medicalization has ascended in influence over birth and motherhood. Rewriting the Mother Code must include strengthening your ability to listen to your inner voice, often called intuition.

Intuition can be described in several ways, but the definition of it as a "feeling of knowing without being able to say how one knows," which the Root-Bernsteins use in their book *Sparks of Genius,*[2] is a rather succinct and incisive definition. I call it our inner voice, though it can be influenced by outer wisdom. The separation of women on the verge of giving birth from other women in a typical hospital setting—including and perhaps especially other women who are themselves mothers—ends up desacralizing the event. In many environments, society has marginalized the unique spheres of feminine knowledge and wisdom.

Strengthening your intuition builds the power you hold in the world, and the best way to build it is to listen to it. One of the best times to follow your intuition is during conception, pregnancy, and the early years of raising children. In a male-dominated society, a woman listening to that inner voice is performing a radical act. This is ironic, considering how many men who are famous for their intellectual and creative work credit intuition as a critical part of the process of problem-solving. Still, women's intuition as an inferior, overly emotional form of reasoning is a recurring trope in modern society.

These apparent contradictions make sense when one considers that a double standard between genders has been part of our society's agenda for centuries. It is a recurring presence in the Mother Code. Men aren't opposed to intuition, but there is a clear reluctance to accept women as intellectual equals. Because intuition involves understanding that seems to precede logic, it can be categorized as emotional or impulsive and fed into the narrative that women are irrational. At the same time, men in the fields of

---

2 Root-Bernstein, Robert Scott, and Michele Root-Bernstein. *Sparks of Genius: The Thirteen Thinking Tools of the World's Most Creative People.* Houghton Mifflin Harcourt, 2001, 2.

science, mathematics, and the arts have known all along that it is a critical part of their processes. This is only a contradiction if one expects the playing field to be level and fair.

Your intuition is your guide through a process that many of your advisors in a typical American birth will either never experience or have not yet experienced. You are the expert in many, many aspects of how your body is changing. Trust yourself—no one understands what you are going through more than you do, no matter how many people try to tell you otherwise. If you can choose the team supporting you through your pregnancy and birth, make sure it is a diverse group. Insist that women are among the deciders where you may not be able to make decisions for yourself. And let no one tell you that you must tolerate disrespect.

In her book, *37 Seconds: Dying Revealed Heaven's Help—A Mother's Journey*, Stephanie Arnold shares the lack of respect and unwillingness of doctors, friends, and even her husband to acknowledge her profound and tragic "seeing" of the upcoming birth of her child. Call it a premonition, a vision, a window into the future, her intuitive and real experience of what was to come was rejected by all but one caregiver—her anesthesiologist. Had this woman not joined her in her sensing of what was to come, Stephanie would not have come back from her 37-second flatline, and she would have died. Sadly, until Stephanie's story is part of the curriculum in medical school, it will remain a paranormal or new-age tale.

Our ability to capture the insight gleaned from a woman's intuition is critical in this work. It is a crucial aspect of making the leap from the outdated Mother Code to the new framework in which a mother's development is seen as central to our larger worldview. Intuition is complicated to the linear mind, but it is by no means illogical or unscientific. There is an active discussion in scholarly journals about ways to increase its use in medical and scientific contexts.

Intuition has an important role to play in Rewriting the Mother

Code in part because the task at hand includes thinking outside of patterns ingrained in us for years. Fortunately, this is a mission for which mothers are uniquely equipped. Everyone can rewire their brains, but the key to success in that effort is neuroplasticity. But pregnancy triggers changes in the brain that dramatically increase the plasticity of the mind. The best time to start rewriting your Mother Code is right now. The period during which your mind will be most receptive to such transformational efforts is from the moment you are pregnant forward.

This is exciting news! Unfortunately, this time when you are most open to change and even transformation, you are overwhelmed with the newness of it all, so our tendency is toward the safe route of what is known and comfortable. There is no shame in that, but if you don't even know it is possible to benefit from this opportunity for a brain-wiring reboot that will pay off in dividends later, you could miss it. However, if you plan in advance for it and seek support from supportive allies to create a *culture* of transformation, your chances at successfully rewiring your brain increase significantly.

Culture
Motherhood is more deeply woven into our lives than may be apparent at first glance. We have our relationship to our own mother and our children to consider. But we are also influenced by the entirety of our upbringing, including the presence (or, in some cases, an equally significant absence) of the mother or someone (or ones) representing the mother. In every period, in every society, culture drives what is considered to be good and bad. It is the meaning within the zeitgeist, the general feeling that people have about any number of topics, from the banal to the big defining issues of society. Everything happening is a part of the cultural construct and reinforces the system we operate within, whether we know it or not.

Moving beyond that system is not a small matter. It is not

unusual for people to see themselves as rebelling against society only to realize later that they were a part of reinforcing the culture all along. True transformation requires a deep understanding of the cultural subject matter which one wishes to redefine. Motherhood is as rooted a concept as any other in every single collection of humans. Mothers are programmed with a set of myths that everyone in the society also understands to be tremendously important—in many cases, even sacred. One does not simply reject a whole worldview that has been woven into one's very consciousness.

A principle of physics known as the Observer Effect essentially states that experiments with particles are changed by someone watching the experiment. We can imagine, for example, a woman who realizes that the rules she has been made to internalize, such as the limits of mothers, the expectation of servitude, and the selfishness of wanting to grow from the experience, are not her ideas. All of that has been programmed inside of her—the Mother Code. Once she becomes aware that she does not have to be a part of the experiment but can instead define it herself if she will take the necessary steps to do so, she becomes the observer instead of a particle. And for her, once she begins to free herself, her experience of culture relative to the Mother Code begins to change as well.

In becoming the observer, you can know that there is a chance at freedom from a system that makes motherhood a prison and a position of servitude. It becomes clear that, through a willingness to be open to seeing the world as it is, you can write your own version of that code. This new code can prioritize you and the people you care about instead of a system that makes its own perpetuation the highest end.

Seeing the Mother Code everywhere without having to force it is a sign that you have reached a deep level of mindful observation. Dismantling the power the existing Mother Code has over you will ultimately necessitate the creation of a new Code.

Cultivating an ongoing awareness denotes a Mother Code fluency which means you are ready to systematically take that burdensome cultural construct apart.

We will rebuild together, just as we will learn to see together. I hope that in the not-too-distant future, women choosing motherhood will look back in utter disbelief that we could survive within a cultural system that good mothers go it alone with minimal or little support. And worse, we would defend this badge of honor and decorously accept the ultimate title of Super Mom. Our future selves will laugh at the silliness and absurdity and cry tears of compassion for the pain we endured when shifting the culture.

Let us hear the rallying cry of our future sisters to stand, sit, and dance in community. Let us correct the overswing of the pendulum that took us away from our tribes, away from tight-knit families, and open spaces and put us alone in tiny boxes where we could do it all (by ourselves). Now that we know the realities and have experienced the extremes of each end of the pendulum, we are invited to envision a harmonious culture of community. We can build a culture that is rooted in empowering every individual to maximize their gifts and potential for the greater good of the community.

Let yourself imagine the possibilities of motherhood where you are safe, secure, and lifted up. We are creating that culture as we envision it collectively. Now it is not a matter of *if* it will happen but *when* and how wonderful it will be!

Engage

It is one thing to study music theory and the anatomy of our vocal cords and how they work, but at some point, the only way to understand the voice is to sing! Putting VOICE into action and engaging with each aspect is when the concert starts. It is as raucous as it is peaceful. It is as wild as it is sublime. Instead of running in circles grasping at an impossible cultural directive, you can engage with clarity and purpose.

You will know you are making purposeful and transformational noise when people—our families and strangers alike—start to directly challenge you and try to curtail and even put a gag over your mouth to stop you from using your VOICE. It is understandable to have some trepidation. It can be messy and there are consequences when you use your voice to have the mothering experience you want to have. But it's worth it to see the benefits of engaging in something mindful or something you were afraid to try and then feeling exhilarated afterward that you took the leap.

As with any courageous quest, I expect you to be hesitant to engage fully in using your VOICE to rewrite your Mother Code—even though you cognitively understand it and you know it will benefit you. We all *know* we should get plenty of sleep, exercise, and eat well, but it doesn't mean we do it all the time. I know that I feel my best and have the most energy when I leave refined sugar, gluten, and dairy out of my diet, exercise regularly, and get seven to eight hours of sleep a night. And I know I am not a flawed or bad person if I choose to have a piece (or two or three) of pizza, miss a workout, and stay up late binge-watching a show. Yes, I am conscious of the choice I am making to feel bloated and lethargic. I am at my best when I remember my vision for my body as a vessel of spirit and pleasure. I have loads of energy when I own my choice at the moment and tune into my body and what it really needs versus what it wants. And still, sometimes, I just need a break!

Understanding what the Code looks and sounds like is both complex and simple. We already know that there are problems with the way people think and talk about being a mother. But peeling away the layers that cloud our understanding and then knowing what to do about it will take a little work. Or a lot of work. You get to choose! The good news is that no matter how much time and energy you put into this process, you will be rewarded with perspectives that can alter your experience of mothering in positive and meaningful ways. In Part Three, we will spend lots of time exploring how to fully engage with and live your rewritten Mother Code and what it can look like in your life.

A commitment to engaging in practices that will deepen one's understanding and rewire our programming is important in securing sustained self-actualized outcomes in our mothering experience. And when we do, we engage in life with eyes wide open from a place of curiosity, shifting old beliefs and behaviors, attending workshops or finding an effective coach, and connecting with other people who are likewise engaged in rewriting their Mother Code in their own lives.

Patience, compassion, and intention are qualities we want to foster as we engage in the adventure of rewriting our Mother Codes. The good news is you have already engaged in at least two practices. It was your curiosity and yearning for a cosmic experience of mothering that led you to this book. You have read the pages leading to this one. Congratulations! Celebrate yourself!

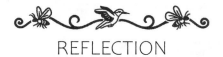

REFLECTION

Whether it be the sound of your voice or all that is in the VOICE framework, reflect on how you have used your voice to experience pleasure. If you cannot think of any right away, take a moment to consider it now.

How might you use your voice to ask for that which is only for your pleasure?

Is there a joyous sound to be made for something you accomplished recently?

Can you recall a memory that inspires pleasure and give voice to it?

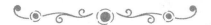

I feel secure in this moment that claiming my VOICE played a significant role in rewriting my Mother Code. In whatever ways we partner with Spirit to create our reality, our voice matters.

Rich and I created a *vision* for our conception journey. Rather than feel victimized or succumb to options that would have come more out of fear than discernment, I took *ownership* of my body by expanding my knowledge and raising my awareness of all the forces at play in this vulnerable space of conception. I used my *intuition* to guide me in chartering unknown territory, giving equal weight to my emotional responses *and* my rational thinking. Through this I was creating my *culture* of community. Rather than stay alone in the process as would have been my historical inclination, I asked directly for support from my doctor friend. We garnered the loving support of a diverse group of people on our pilgrimage, and while I have not mentioned it directly, I included spirit and unseen guides in my community as well. There were many times through this part of my mothering journey I felt scared, hopeless, and lost, but I continued to *engage.*

To be honest, sometimes it meant engaging with my doubts and fears to weed out the mistaken beliefs about myself and what I could expect from the world to get to what were real issues to be contended with. If you make choices guided by your values that shift your life course even one degree from your reflexive programming, you will move in a different direction. Making intuitive and discerned choices has the power to take us further and further from the limited norms of our families and culture. It is possible when we use our VOICE.

Your success in this endeavor hangs on your level of engagement. It's circular and not linear. You will use your intuition; you will create a community. They will support you, and then you will engage fully and then guess what—your experience of life will change. So, what happens then? Well, you go back to vision and start all over again because your vision may have expanded. It will always expand because when you use your VOICE, you transform, your perspective stretches, and you see more possibilities you couldn't see before.

Whether you are ready to be curious from a distance, put your toe in the water, or dive into the deep end, it doesn't matter. The only thing that matters is you being present to yourself and choosing your path. It is tuning into and using your VOICE that will provide the pathway and guidance you need. It is remembering you always have many choices. It is remembering that no expert, no family member, no friend surpasses the *vision* of your mothering journey. You *own* your authority and experience. You follow your *intuition* for the embodied experience you know is possible. You create a *culture* of community that supports your vision. You *engage* in every part of your process with all of your emotions.

Rite of Passage—First Trimester

Congratulations! You completed your first trimester of Rewriting the Mother Code! And just as every pregnancy is unique to each woman, your journey in these first three chapters is yours to honor and explore. For some, it may have been smooth sailing physically, but emotionally, you were triggered right and left. For others, like nausea and tiredness that can knock you off your feet, what we have discussed in this first section may have done the same. It is dizzying and stomach-churning to have our beliefs and sacred cows poked at. Like organs starting to move around in our body to make room for your baby, you may have had discomfort as you stretched into expanding your thinking.

The first trimester of physical pregnancy is a time of profound transformation, most of which is unseen. A fertilized egg is now a rapidly dividing cluster of cells that has embedded itself in your uterine lining and has begun to develop into an embryo. By the time the first month has passed, the neural tube, which will become the brain and spinal cord, is already forming. Another heart begins to beat inside of you, and the tiny buds that will later grow into arms and legs begin to appear. As organs like the liver and kidneys take shape, the embryo transitions into a fetus, and although it's only about the size of a pea, it's growing at an incredible pace.

You are not merely the host of this miracle in the making; you are having a parallel experience. So much growth and discerned decision-making have brought you to this stage of your development. The egg of your desire to mother another human and the intention you put forth to have it be so has imbedded itself within you. Your dream begins to reflect physical reality. It is a vulnerable and precarious time when everything is new. Tender little buds of this new version of you are taking shape. Your senses and emotions are heightened and unfiltered. Your awareness expands, and the potential for transforming outdated circuitry into wiring that resonates with your voice is open and available to you. An additional musical note adds to the rhythmic drumming of your beating heart. The second trimester is where even more growth and transformation take place. You see and feel yourself expanding. The fetus becomes very real as it knocks and kicks at your belly. Nature takes its course, but your Mother Code will inform how you experience it and continue to transform through it.

PART TWO

SECOND TRIMESTER

Crowned by a rainbow of my becoming.
I sit in awe and wonder of
the alchemy of elements
that create this beauty.
A mystical gift that can be explained by science,
but why ruin the fun.
When the unseen shows itself,
bends itself, into
a circle of
red
orange
yellow
green
blue
indigo.
Reflecting all that is true,
all that is possible for

our radiant being
Stretching around eternity.
Into the everything.

Connecting, bridging, mixing
The invisible made visible
In the air.

Chapter 4

Motherhood is a Prism

"Look over there! Do you see it?" I yelled with excitement to my husband, who was driving us along the coastal road of Maui, Hawaii.

"See what?" he replied, a little annoyed as my sudden outburst took him by surprise.

"The rainbow! Over there! You can see the whole thing!" I pointed out the window toward the landscape on our left.

"Wow!" we said in unison, marveling at the glory and wonder of the sight.

"Turn down that road ahead!" I demanded.

"What? Why?" he asked annoyed to be told what to do, but did so, being accustomed to my antics.

"It looks so close...let's see if we can touch it?!" I said with childlike enthusiasm. I knew that it was impossible, but I was compelled to try.

What is it about a rainbow that evokes such awe and draws us toward it? I am sure you can recount a similar experience. Whether it's one large arch over a body of water or shards of color scattered across the floor and up the wall of a room, spotting the red, orange, yellow, green, blue, indigo, and violet of refracted light never ceases to delight. Even in my grumpiest moments, this band of color has the power to shift my mood, if even for a few seconds. The dialogue I shared above is universal and common, but it is never ordinary because seeing a rainbow strikes something deep inside of us that is powerful and calls us to touch the awe and wonder of visible transformation.

Now, imagine that *you* are a prism. Whether you are made of crystal or glass, a raindrop or a waterfall, you are beautiful just as you are, and the world is made more beautiful with you in it. You are whole and complete, and nothing needs to change about you.

You may choose, or not, to explore more about this already perfect being that you are. Should you decide to step toward self-prism awareness, you will discover that when you shine light on yourself, magic happens. A rainbow of colors emanates from YOU! Wow! Did you know this spectrum of vibrant colors was hidden inside of you? Wanting more and more of your colors to be revealed, you notice that some areas of your prism are covered, blocking the light from entering. As the light blockers of childhood and cultural wiring are identified and removed, your radiance is dispersed even more expansively. You are delighted with the discovery of your true colors being revealed. This is the light of universal truth and authentic awareness.

Knowing you are one with the beauty around you and that you yourself are as breathtaking as a sunset, as much of a miracle as an ocean—incredibly, this is only part of the journey of discovery. Rewriting your Mother Code unfolds a new reality, and it opens the door to an even closer relationship with the light. You will go from being aware of your miraculous self to also manifesting that miracle of light at will and even sow the seeds of that miracle within others.

Now that you have raised your awareness of this power and potential inside of you, anything is possible. You have choices you didn't know you had before. Your first choice to consider is whether to *view* the prism simply as a pretty crystal that makes rainbows or *experience* the prism as a portal. The choice is yours.

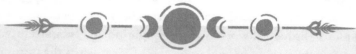

SUN RITUAL

The sun's energy travels across the universe before its warm rays come to rest on your face or light up water molecules to create a rainbow. It is a wondrous ball of fiery gases that has both the power to sustain life as well as destroy it. Your mother energy is similarly wondrous in its capacity to be life-giving and respected for its power.

As the first light of day begins to glow, find a quiet place where you can face the rising sun. Stand tall with your feet firmly grounded, and close your eyes. Breathe deeply, feeling or imagining the warmth of the sun as it touches your face. With each breath, imagine the golden light filling your heart, infusing you with strength and warmth. Stretch your arms wide, embracing the sun as if gathering its energy into your being.

Whisper softly to yourself, "I am a source of light, warmth, and love for myself, my family, and my friends."

Let this energy settle in your heart, carrying it with you throughout the day as a reminder of your inner strength and nurturing spirit.

Motherhood is a Portal

When you open yourself to receive the light, magic happens. You can bend light. The prism offers you all types of dimensions; some you see only fleetingly, others we see with more certainty. Depending on how the light bends, you have a different view. You don't know how you will see or understand your experience until you look through the prism of your upbringing, circumstances, cultures, etc. Trying to hold to one set of ideas when the prism is so diverse will only leave you feeling like you are wrong when you don't reflect the colors you think you are supposed to. And sometimes, the light bends when we least expect it.

Let's assume that anything that touches you from the outside is light. Imagine that anything, anyone, any circumstance, or any programming you receive can be transformed into rainbows of light. Unlike actual prisms that require a literal light, you have the choice to receive *everything* as light. To go a step further, let's exchange the word light with truth. Think broadly about the implications of this. The truth of your experience, the truth that hurts, the feedback that only has 1% of actual truth all contain the properties needed to create beauty and wonder.

St. Teresa of Avila, a 14th-century mystic and Catholic saint, was known to say that a good day for her was a day in which she received a humbling truth.[1] To take it a step further, even if she felt 99% of what the person was sharing wasn't accurate, that 1% held a potent beam of truth. If you are anything like me, receiving feedback or direct criticism is something I find challenging, and I often meet it with defensiveness. Not St. Teresa! The humbling truth allowed her to grow personally, which she felt brought her closer to God. To be clear, she isn't saying a good day is one where

---

1 I recommend Mirabai Starr's excellent treatment of St. Theresa: Starr, Mirabai. *Saint Teresa of Avila: Passionate Mystic.* Sounds True, 2013. There is a thorough essay on St. Theresa's dedication to humility at https://carmeliteinstitute.net/teresa-of-avila-living-a-life-of-humility/.

she levitates in ecstatic rapture or has divine communion with Jesus, which she also experienced regularly. Instead, it was receiving a truth that would let her know herself, and she believed that the more she knew herself, the more she would know God. I find this inspiring and challenging.

What happens inside the prism when light enters is the refraction—the alchemy of the transformation. You, too, are a vessel of transformation. It may not always be as instantaneous because we have not evolved enough to make it instantaneous, but we have that capacity. So, for now, you must do the work. The work starts with opening yourself to the light as we have now defined it. Once you open to the light, you receive everything that comes your way as data. That data can be an awareness, a piece of feedback, a compliment, a criticism, a traumatic event, or an achievement. You have the choice with them all to bend the light and choose your reaction. For example, bending the light is to take that information or interaction, identify the pain point from your past that is triggered, release the stuck emotions you kept inside because it wasn't safe in the past to feel them, and finally experience cathartic healing through that process.

Contained within every choice we make, every circumstance we encounter, wanted or not, on our mothering journey is a rainbow of possibilities. Whether you realize it or not, simply by getting this far, you have become much more aware of the framework that has informed your understanding of motherhood your whole life.

One way our most basic coding remains intact is through its invisibility: We rarely think to question why we have a bunch of assumptions about mothering, or if we do, we conclude that it is natural or instinct. (This, too, is part of the code by the way—the message that the code itself is an intrinsic part of our identity). By engaging with me in questioning that framework, you are not only revealing your true colors but also seeing the world in a new way.

This is *your* project. I am laying out how the code operating within can limit you and how to overcome that, but the specifics are up to you. This is to give you the power to decide how your future—and your family's—will look. So, pick and choose!

On the quest to identify your own Mother Codes, I encourage you to make the following agreements:

Agree to stay out of victimhood.

Agree to avoid parental blame.

Agree to avoid cultural blame.

Also, consider that the Mother Code you operate with exists beyond good and evil and taken altogether, the Code is intended to perpetuate a system that is important to keep society functioning. We have reached a stage of development where we recognize that some of these elements are harmful to people, but that doesn't mean a cabal of evildoers came up with a malicious operating system and disseminated it like a virus.

You have a different vision of the world, and you can override the elements that don't further your growth as a person, but we can do so without internalizing a sense of some malicious force at play in our lives. It is probably easier to dispassionately disregard those messages we no longer consider valid and reinforce a new code rather than pouring anger into the old Code.

It can feel intense, tedious, and even overwhelming sometimes, but it is a precious and courageous undertaking. You will have feelings. Embrace them! Your emotions are your guide. They confirm your reality, and they are the antidote to victimhood and blame. Trust them and even when you don't have words or memories, your emotions are revealing your story.

How We Reflect Our Choices

You came here to Earth for a purpose. You chose your mother's womb as a launching pad for your life. Remember, you picked this specific human experience. This is YOUR human experience, and no one can dictate it. Yet so many try to dictate it to you, and the Mother Code itself operates as a sort of self-regulator in which the worldview of others is imposed on you from within. As we unravel these instances of assumption and presupposition, I hope that you will find some pleasure in putting what you truly think and feel in the place of that indoctrination. On this path of reflection, your true face is the treasure.

One of the places I see the unconscious mind at work is when a woman is asked if she wants to have children—now or someday. When I hear replies like "Yes! I have always known I want to have children," or the opposite, "No, I know I do not want to have children," my curiosity is piqued. Most women will not be questioned further if they say yes, but if they say no, then a whole slew of questions come rolling toward them. "Oh really, why not?" Or "You just haven't found the right partner," or "Don't worry, sweetie, you will change your mind."

This type of interaction reflects our culture and our hard-wiring that all women should have children. We will dig into those codes later in the chapter, so we will not address them at the moment. But I want to open your mind to further exploration anytime we say a definitive no or an unexamined yes to this question.

How is it you came to *know*...? What led you to this surety? The *yes* woman will often respond with, "I just know!" or "I have always known since I was a little girl." I am not dismissing our intuitive senses, of course, but once a woman is willing to dig into this, she will discover there is a lot more to that answer than meets the eye.

Same with the definitive *no* woman. A woman has every right to say no and does not need to explain herself. But this isn't about that. This is about exploring the personal and cultural wiring that leads us to respond unreflectively to questions about a life choice that is so significant.

I find when a woman allows herself to explore this question, the choice she makes has depth and meaning for her. Sometimes, the inquiry does shift a woman's choice one way or the other, but again, that is never the point of the inquiry. It is all about learning about ourselves and making discerned choices.

I realized much later, after having children, that I never asked this question of myself—my journey revealed it for me. I was mentally in yes mode and going with the program, except my body was communicating for me in its resistance to an outcome that resulted in children. My body was saying no when I thought I was saying yes, and not until I dug deep into it did I discover the block.

This is a big question and one you can start exploring now or get into later after you have had a chance to do some digging and being with yourself, uncovering your Mother Codes.

Understanding Where Your Codes Come From

My first master's degree culminated with a capstone project where I wrote and delivered a workshop called, "Your Parents' Marriage or Yours." My husband and I had taken part in a similar workshop some years before, and it was so powerful and enlightening for us that I wanted to build on the learning. The awareness that we will inherently create relationships that mirror our parents and stir up our unfinished business was revelatory. This workshop helped illuminate the impact of two family systems coming together in a way that just talking about it falls short. We used a tool called a genogram. It is similar to a family tree going back to your grandparents (or further if you want), only instead of just names and dates of births and deaths, you fill in as much data as you can find about each person in the family. I recommend *You Can Go Home Again: Reconnecting with Your Family* by Monica McGoldrick and Tracey Laszloffy as an excellent resource for creating your own genogram.

You will be taking note of relationship patterns: divorces, affairs, addictions, education levels, employment, health issues, and longevity, to name a few. Getting information through memory and through interviewing family members makes this a rich exercise. I am a visual person, so seeing it mapped showed patterns through the generations.

I noticed patterns like alcoholism, enmeshed (overly close and disempowering) mother-daughter relationships, affairs, cut-off relationships, low education levels, and undeveloped gifts and talents. I also saw parents giving their children more than they had, longevity on both sides, resilience, living through traumatic experiences, and sobriety. Out of this, I had a sense of the shoulders I was standing on. I realized that the challenges and blocks I had to live my dreams were embedded in these long-standing patterns.

You will probably have some level of discomfort or even triggers and emotional reactions as you go through this practice. It is possible to keep your distance from the feelings and go through it like an exercise. Or, if you want to, you can do deep work on this with a coach or therapist. Remember, you are on a journey of discovery here. You are inviting the data into your prism that will inform your vision for yourself on your mothering journey. The more you can tell the truth about what you see and the impact it has had on your choices, the more you are giving yourself a huge gift and opportunity to bend the light.

The Mother Codes

Every society and culture have their codes, and they are an important part of uniting people, especially people from different backgrounds. In the U.S., we rely on codes like the intentions of the Founding Fathers and a vision of the American Dream to keep people optimistic about who we are as a people and to unite us all under one flag. Likewise, we have ideas about motherhood that feed into the idea of being *e pluribus unum* (out of many, one); despite our varied backgrounds, we can count on some things being the same all over the country, such as good old-fashioned motherhood.

Remember that all codes are created by people. As you look at each code, consider whether it is something you feel strongly about and how you would address the idea behind it. Notice any desire to reject one or more codes. This is normal when confronted with a concept that does not fit the consensual reality. The opportunity before you is to be curious and to consider that, if these are not ultimately empowering truths, what are?

Code #1: *You immediately fall in love with your baby, and you have only blissful love from the moment you hold them. If you are over-whelmed with intense feelings of anxiety or sadness after your child's birth, there is something wrong with you.*

How did it come to be that a woman is expected to have this specific experience, and if she doesn't, she has failed? Birthing a baby is work. It is powerful and intense work. Given the intensity of the experience and the uniqueness of every birth, can we show some grace?

Maybe your labor was so intense for you that feeling anything beyond the exhaustion or even trauma for some time was all you could do. Maybe the overall elation of the experience has you tuning into yourself and the feelings you are having. Or maybe for no particular reason, you just don't have that moment.

Millions, if not billions, of other moms have had that same experience, and everything turned out just fine. That self-inflicted pressure or judgment is self-defeating and even violent to yourself.

Do you remember when I told you about my dinner with my daughter and her friend, whose mother instantly bonded with her when she was born? And how I admitted that this didn't happen to me? In its retelling, this may sound like a bravely honest moment or something you could never have a conversation about with your children, but at the moment, I was just expressing myself. I wasn't trying to stick to some high ideals or make a philosophical point. I was telling my daughter something true about me that maybe wasn't what she wanted to hear, but it was the truth, and I want her to know what's real about her life, not a fantasy version of it.

Understanding and normalizing the many potential reactions, emotions, and bonding experiences is essential for the well-being of the birthing person. The last thing anyone needs at such a significant transition is to feel the pressure to perform or have any prescribed reaction.

Rewrite the Code: A mother's first experience of holding her baby is a sacred event, however it happens and whatever feelings arise from it. You have the experience you need to have for the life you are living.

There is a vicious circle in mothering literature in which negative thoughts related to being a mother are considered outside of normal behavior. If you try to figure out when it's okay to be dissatisfied with being a mother or how much sluggishness is normal, the answer is never and none. I am here to tell you that it's okay to have the full range of emotions and reactions throughout your entire mothering experience. You will love, hate, cherish, and even regret motherhood sometimes. To think we may only talk about the good stuff leaves out the richness and fullness of the experience. It is also an unfair burden to put on a mother, to expect her to stuff down the not-so-picture-perfect moments, hours, or days or to assume that the pictures we see on social media reflect the full truth of the experience.

Several years ago, a woman published a column in a paper about regretting having children.[2] The reaction was overwhelming. She received huge amounts of hate mail, much of it stating that there was something wrong with her because she regretted being a mother. Somehow, we have reached a point in our society where expressing hatred to a stranger because they have a view you don't agree with is considered normal, but regretting a decision you made that changed your life unalterably is not.

Feel your feelings—they are yours. When it is suggested that you use medication to deal with strong feelings, be discerning.

2 You can read this piece at https://www.dailymail.co.uk/femail/article-2303588/The-mother-says-having-children-biggest-regret-life.html#comments.

Pain is sometimes a sign of growth. The optimal solution to experiencing feelings, including sadness, regret, and anger, is to get to the source of those feelings and learn from them. It can feel really scary to do this in a culture that quickly wants you to mask your feelings so you can "do your job" as a mother.

Rewrite the Code: When a mother feels overwhelmed with anxiety or sadness, this is probably an important inflection point in her journey to be valued, examined, and excavated. It should not be buried, nor should the mother feel shame for having strong feelings.

Code #2: *Always put the needs of your children first, and you will be a good mother, and your children will turn out fine. Your needs come after everyone else's now, including those of your spouse or partner, because your child is your top source of ongoing joy and fulfillment from here on out.*

Being a mama bear protecting her cubs is a powerful image. Come anywhere near them, and you will be sorry! But we seem to exclude the pictures that make up the bulk of the day in the life of a mama bear and her cubs—sleeping when and where she wants, eating when she is hungry, and letting her cubs fall down and learn. Sometimes, a child's needs *should* come first. But mom is a human being who has equally important needs. Let's learn to be honest and distinguish between cultural messaging that dictates servitude and all-consuming mindsets over creating space for quality time with your children and with yourself.

To take it a step further, I aspire to the adage, "If mama isn't happy, nobody is happy." Your nourishment, self-care, sense of well-being, and affirmation lead to a person who has the energy and desire to care for her family.

Many of us come from families where our mothers' and grandmothers' needs were not considered or honored, and their labor was exploited. The language that asked women what they felt and needed was not spoken in our mothers' and grandmothers' day. And because this emotional language is missing, our mothers and grandmothers did not learn how to speak to it. They did not know how to ask themselves what they felt and needed or how to share their trauma. And they did not know how to teach their daughters how to honor their feelings and needs.

There is a term for this kind of disconnection from a mother and her needs. Rosjke Hasseldine calls it "The Culture of Female Service."[3] It is a term she uses to cover all the cultural beliefs that we have about how women are the nurturers and that it is a woman's role and duty to serve her family and community without needing care in return. This mindset has created the generational pattern of women's unacknowledged needs. It has created a pattern of self-neglect that our mothers and grandmothers learned to tolerate and normalize because they did not know anything different.

Rewrite the Code: The more a mother sees her well-being and that of her children as the same, the healthier and stronger all the people who make up the family will be.

A spouse or partner viewing the needs of children as most important is often an incorrect assumption. Using a traditional heterosexual couple as an example, even when Dad thinks that Mom should put the kids ahead of her own needs, he does not necessarily think the same thing about his own needs. In fact, it is often the case that mothers are torn in two directions by partners who want them to prioritize children over everything and prioritize the partners over everything, too. If that sounds impossible, it's because it is. Humans have no firm commitment to rationality when receiving care.

So, first, partners don't necessarily agree that children should come first all the time—even when they say they do. Second, even

---

3 Hasseldine discusses this phenomenon in detail at https://www.rosjke.com/wp-content/uploads/2016/11/policyreviewRosjke.pdf.

when it's clear that a child has a top-priority need, not all partners are going to see that or act accordingly if they do. People can be selfish. And we can miss very obvious things—especially when seeing them interfere with what we want. This code sets mothers up for expectations about adults that don't square with reality.

Rewrite the Code: Honoring everyone's desires equally creates harmony and a mutually loving environment. Consistent communication about everyone's needs minimizes unexpected disagreements and prevents crossed wires.

My daughters *have* been a source of joy and fulfillment, to be sure, and those relationships are only getting richer and more meaningful over time. I cherish them. They are also very frustrating. I am sometimes angry, sad, disappointed, and simply fed up.

Children are human beings. We are *supposed* to have complicated relationships, and the sign of that is a relationship that lets the full range of emotions be expressed. That's how being human works. It will be unsettling and messy, and you will need support to navigate everything that gets churned up when you invite authenticity into your motherhood. And it's just as true in their twos and threes as it is in their twenties and thirties. It's okay not to find perfect bliss in every moment with them.

Rewrite the Code: Your feelings for your children are complex and deeply felt.

Code #3: *Don't worry about maintaining your own identity. You have a new one that really matters—being a mother. Being a mother is your primary way to feel worth as a human.*

Phew, this is a big one! How do we encompass this transformative experience of becoming a mother and not overidentify with it? It takes claiming, appreciating, and understanding who you are outside of motherhood first and then adding this element into the mix. It doesn't make you any more whole or matter any more than you did before you had a child.

Rewrite the Code: Motherhood is something I incorporate into my wholeness and becomes an additional facet of my identity.

Having a mom who expected that she would be perpetually affirmed by her children and having a happy childhood are not the same thing. It's like treating children as though they are antidepressants. It puts impossible pressure on the relationship between child and parent and imposes on moms yet another way to be disappointed in themselves.

There is another window we can open to see into our childhoods and family systems and the effect they have on us. It takes the data from the genogram and guides us to see the possible impact of the patterns on our lives. Families create stories or codes about their culture. Mostly, these stories are a way to deal with pain and anxiety in the family, and they become the shadow on our prisms that block the light of truth. These stories have tremendous power over us until we face them head-on. You do that by identifying the beliefs and rules that got wired in because of the story.

Something I appreciated about my childhood was that my mother owned a children's clothing store. It was called Pepi's, and I loved it because I started working there while I was in grade school. On the surface, all of that was great. One of the *codes* regarding my mom's role in the business was hearing my father tell my mother that it was fine for her to have the store as a hobby but don't show a profit because he didn't want to pay taxes on the income. Out of that code, I internalized the *belief* that women only have hobbies, that men do serious work and provide for the family, and to keep your success small or you will get in trouble. And then a couple of the *rules* include don't be successful as a woman and do depend on a man for your survival.

Think about phrases or sayings your family used. I also find it useful to look for the codes, beliefs, and rules in various areas of life.

These can include but are not limited to self, work/career, money, relationships (family of origin, friends, family of creation), sex, spirituality, and community. The point is to cover as much ground in the way your family operated as you can. You may find that a pattern emerges or a core belief that carried through them all.

This can start to get pretty raw, and more likely, you are finding it challenging to keep it an intellectual exercise. The distance between the historical data and the emotions they evoke is narrowing. This is a good time to have lots of compassion and an even better time to celebrate all this work you have done so far. Even if you are not writing them down, just thinking about these family dynamics is stirring the pot inside of you.

Rewrite the Code: Growing into the best version of yourself in all seasons of your life is a valuable source of affirmation, and raising children can be an integral part of that growth.

Code #4: Being a mother is an innate skill. You will automatically know how to do it. And when you feel insecure and doubt yourself as a mother, follow the guidance of experts or your mother or close family members.

You are coming to motherhood (or have arrived!) with a number of strengths that will serve you well, and additional strengths are waiting for you to unlock them. But you do not have a built-in set of instructions.

This idea is a setup for failure—or at least to keep you constantly insecure because you did not automatically know how to be a mother from day one. Ironically, the same society that will make you think you are deficient if you don't already know things you never learned also tells you to trust experts who will instruct you how to be a mother when it comes to things you already know. These elements are closely related. By setting the bar impossibly high and then telling you to turn your decision-making over to experts if you can't clear it, society is setting you up to be an unthinking babysitting machine.

We all have things we liked and didn't like about our childhoods, and they form the basis of our knowledge of being a mother. Think about the modeling of mothering that you saw every day through your parents and other adults. What are their behaviors telling you about how people ought to behave when raising children?

One way I suggest engaging with this question and becoming your own expert is by listing what you *liked* and what you *didn't like* about your upbringing and how you were parented. Put "Childhood" at the top and likes and dislikes in two columns. Remember this is not a list of good and bad practices, though your opinions of the integrity of things you saw or that happened to you as a child are important and valid.

Keeping the columns about what we liked or didn't like helps keep it more neutral and lets you include more items—maybe you hated Sunday dinner when your aunt and uncle came over, but you don't know why—trust it and write it down, exclude nothing. No explanations are necessary here. Include as much as you are moved to add to the list.

Here are examples to get you started…

Likes: my mother wanted to have children; my mother owned a children's clothing store while I was growing up; my grandparents would live with us two to three months of the summer; we lived in a lovely home on a shipping channel; my mom went on buying trips for the store with her business partner…

Dislikes: my mom relied on us for her emotional needs: I never saw my parents hold hands or show affection; a traditional family structure where the dad made the money and the mom took care of everything related to the children; even though the mom worked, it was just for enjoyment and not a career; she gave birth with pain medication; did not breastfeed…

Now, what should we do with this list? The first thing to consider is that everything on that list, no matter how seemingly insignificant, has real power. The fact that you have made the association means it has taken root in your mind. *Rewrite the Code: Being a mother is a call to lifelong learning and personal development.*

If you ever doubt that your voice is powerful, reflect for a moment on how much energy is put into silencing it. Our society is deeply intimidated by the intelligence of the feminine. And it's no surprise! A culture based on making people feel inferior, the use of force, hierarchies, and isolating individualism is going to reject competing views that are inclusive, reconciling, nonviolent, and communal.

Learn to listen to your own VOICE! The journey toward rewriting your Mother Code is not just a means to an end; developing the skills it takes to do the work gets you most of the way there. The purpose woven into bringing new life into the world is to strengthen all life, including your own. When you can't hear yourself, don't begin by assuming you are not worth hearing. Listen more closely.

Rewrite the Code: When you feel insecure and doubt yourself as a mother, find a space in which you can listen to yourself more clearly and take the time you need to hear what you have to say.

Code #5: *Motherhood provides a supportive nonjudgmental network of other mothers who will help you be the best mother you can be. Automatic sisterhood!*

I love the idea of a vast community of moms looking out for and supporting one another. I work in this field with the idea of building that very community. But I work to build it because it barely exists. Our Western culture isolates mothers. It is a lonely vocation, made even more isolating when juggling other major roles in our lives while also raising children.

The darker truth is our culture further isolates mothers by pitting us against each other. We are living with imposed, unrelenting standards of doing motherhood perfectly, which is impossible, but we are told it is possible so the only way we can feel a modicum of OK-ness is to judge other mothers. When we are going about the most Yin (feminine) activities with the values of the Yang (masculine) values, it is no surprise that cooperation and community get overridden by a competitive, every-woman-for-herself mentality.

So, the more we are willing to tell the truth about our challenges and say the unsayable to each other, the more trust we will build among each other. The clearer I am in my own choices on my mothering journey, the more I can honor other women's, even when they differ from mine.

Rewrite the Code: The more raw and real I am about my mothering journey, the more I will contribute to building a community of mutual support.

To gain clarity on how the motherhood culture has affected and continues to affect you and how you are participating in it, I suggest making another set of lists of what you like and don't like about the culture of being a mother—like you did for your childhood.

This list can include past and current culture.

Some will be both a like and a dislike. For example, I *like* that mothers can find community online, and I *dislike* that it has created its own exclusivity. I mostly see it as a blessing that when my children were babies and for a chunk of raising them, the internet was not something at our disposal. In fact, Facebook was not available to the public until 2006, when my oldest daughter was 10 years old. It doesn't mean some of the same behavior wasn't happening.

The only way you had community with other mothers was to attend or organize playgroups or sign up for "mommy and me"-type-classes. It soon became clear that not every group was created equal or that I would immediately sync with every group I attended. There were cliques, competitiveness, comparing, and complaining. I had my feelings hurt on several occasions because, well, I just didn't fit in with the culture of that group. But when I did find a group or mommy-baby class that had little to none of that, it was heaven and I immersed in some much-needed mama community time.

If you get stuck, some places to look for perspectives on the cultural portrayal of motherhood are movies, TV shows, and social media. Do some internet research specifically on motherhood culture—which will bring up a mere 1.4 billion results for you to peruse. You will also soon notice that the space is dominated by white motherhood culture because in America, the word mother most commonly means *white* mother. Definitely on my dislike list!

It is time to put your research cap on again and do some digging. While you're at it, take a peek at other eras or even cultures of motherhood. You may find things we have left behind you can add to your like list. For example, in Latin America, there is a long-held tradition for the postpartum period they call *la cuarentena*.[4] The custom holds that for forty days following the birth of a child, the birthing person and baby do not leave the house and instead spend that time bonding and healing. I dislike U.S. culture that expects women to bounce back quickly after giving birth. I do like the practice of forty days of mother and baby being taken care of by family and friends or a paid doula.

It can be challenging, but do your best to refrain from judgment and superiority and simply name what you like and don't like without explaining. This work will help you gain clarity on where your judgments of yourself and others and how they mother come from. I also hope it provides compassion for what you are up against in your quest to create an empowering tribe of support around you.

---

4   Here's a summary of the tradition with suggestions on how to adapt it
    to modern life: https://www.babycenter.com/baby/postpartum-health/
    bringing-back-the-hispanic-tradition-of-cuarentena-after-chi_10346386.

Rewrite the Code: The more I understand my own biases and where I am operating out of sync with my feminine values, the more inclusivity and nourishing connection with other mothers I will generate.

Code #6: *A mother's fear, hurt, anger, or pain expressed around her children may limit or harm their development. Likewise, never argue with your spouse or partner in front of your child or children.*

Our society's relationship to acknowledging, identifying, and responsibly expressing strong emotions is so deeply dysfunctional that we have produced more variety and sheer volume of psychotropic medications than any other society in human history. We are desperate to change our minds to change our feelings, yet we have virtually no understanding of the relationship between the heart and the head. The one results directly from the other: How can we know how to influence habits of thinking when the habits of the heart are a mystery to us?

Children will not learn what to do with anger, sadness, or pain if it is hidden from them. So many of us grow up to become adults who do not understand how to deal with our so-called negative feelings and spend the rest of our lives trying to gain a basic understanding of how emotions work! Let your children see you cry. Let them see you in love and in pain, anger, melancholy, embarrassment, joy, and wistfulness. And let them see you share your emotions with personal responsibility.

This is a matter of emotional literacy. What you hide from your children will emerge eventually with their having no understanding of what is happening or how to deal with it. And if you think you can hide these things from them, you are mistaken because they are sensitive beings, and they feel. One of my earliest memories as a child, no more than two years old, was of me standing up in my crib and crying out to my parents. When I sat with this, I had a revelation, which was that I was not crying out to get *myself* tended to, I was crying out because I sensed that *they* needed me.

Through the years, I have not encountered one person who does not have at least some family dysfunction but more often significant trauma in the family line that carries through and often is held in secret. Sometimes, the rules and beliefs around uncovering this trauma are so powerful that merely acknowledging the existence of such matters is unfathomable. I find this especially true in families (like my own) where one of the values is to look good and keep up the appearance of a happy family to the outside world no matter how damaging what is happening behind closed doors is.

Rewrite the Code: Responsibly expressing your fear, hurt, anger, sadness, and joy is a gift to your child. Let children see adults having feelings in safe contexts where they can watch closely, ask questions, and develop some understanding.

Anger deserves special attention because it has a special place in the motherhood codes of our society. "Don't let your children see you fight" is accepted by millions of adults as a truism. But why not? The typical explanation is that it will harm them. This is a good reason to keep your children from seeing horror movies, car accidents, or violent crimes, but these are all outside of the set of experiences that are normal for human beings. Anger is a basic emotion. The problem with hiding anger is that children then don't know what they're feeling when they experience it, or if you have forbidden it, they feel as though they are bad.

A deeper reason parents will hide their anger, which requires a more nuanced approach, is that they cannot control what might happen when they are angry, and it is sometimes extreme. If your fights become physical and lead to cruelty, children should not see or experience that. If you don't know when an argument might get that extreme, you have something to address right away that is probably as pressing as showing your children feelings, if not more so. Anger is a real feeling and should be available in an adult relationship when shared responsibly, but losing all control un-expectedly is a sign of deep and unresolved trauma.

But if you haven't experienced that, don't treat anger as if that's where it leads. Most people, when they become angry, may say unkind things and might even pound a table for emphasis, but there is an understood limit, and that's what children need to see. Feelings can be allowed to flow freely without danger, and we can learn from them. It is also immensely valuable for our children to see conflict resolved. To understand that two people can get angry with each other, take personal responsibility, and move to resolution is priceless.

This is a skill to develop, and I strongly encourage you to take that one on—for your and your children's sake! My husband and I are both conflict avoiders because of growing up in households that expressed anger irresponsibly. Anger showed up as either extreme periodic explosions and/or passive aggressiveness, so in our child logic we were wired with the belief that anger was bad and to be avoided. To build new wiring we consciously practiced having arguments.

Fear is buried for similar reasons, and the approach to letting children see it is much the same. If you are not spiraling out of control when something makes you afraid, then let children know that feeling fear is a normal part of being human. If you have no idea what you might do when something frightens you, start working out where that comes from right away.

Rewrite the Code: It is healthy for children to see their parents argue responsibly and reconcile to have a model of both conflict and its resolution to learn from and refer to.

Code #7: Always hover over your child and watch their every move so you can protect them from experiencing any physical or emotional discomfort or pain. A mother should act as if she doesn't have children at her job and raise her children as if she doesn't have a job.

Imagine for a moment observing the journey a caterpillar takes to become a butterfly. It lives its caterpillar life until, one day, it wraps itself in a cocoon. While in the cocoon, it disintegrates and becomes a gelatinous mass. And then that mass takes a new form, and that new form doesn't fit in the cocoon anymore, so it starts to bust it open. You see it struggling, so you decide to help it out, and you peel off some fibers of the cocoon. Expecting it to take flight, you are surprised to see it limp and motionless. Your attempt to rescue them from their pain and struggle led to them missing out on the critical stage of development, the one in which the struggle brings in vital circulation and helps them build their wing strength.

I heard this analogy in a parenting class, and it struck me deeply. First, it so poignantly exemplifies that there is a line between our help and support contributing and it being debilitating. It is so uncomfortable to see a child struggling, but often, that is more about you than it is about them and what they need. Second, I know firsthand what it is to be shielded from the struggles of life.

I came home from my ballet lesson one day and told my mom I wanted to quit. She said, "Okay." And that was the end of my ballet experience. No inquiry, no asking what the issue was, or even saying finish out the year and we will reassess. I was good at ballet and, from what I recall, I had some easily sort-out-able challenges. The same thing happened with track and softball in high school. On the positive side, she let me know that I can make my own choices. On the negative, and what I consider the debilitating side, is how I didn't develop resilience or fortitude. I didn't have the experience of celebrating sticking with something challenging and getting to the other side. Had I not worked on this in my personal growth, I would have continued that pattern and have a string of things I started and never completed, like getting my doctorate.

This is where parenting reactively can show itself. When we say things like, "I won't do to my child what my parent did to me," it can be for a good reason. But we need to go deeper and resolve that issue for ourselves, so we aren't just doing the opposite of our parents without measuring what is truly the healthiest reaction to each challenge.

Because the personal development of mothers is disregarded in our society, my focus is on rewriting the Mother Code in a way that centers that practice—to benefit the whole family and learn to separate your discomfort from theirs. Let your children work through challenges before you step in. Give them space to feel their feelings and, if at all possible, feel them with them. If they are sad, be sad with them. If their frustration leads to a tantrum, yell and thrash right alongside them. Let them know that it is okay to feel all feelings and let them know you are connected, and what they feel affects you, becomes a part of you.

If you are uncomfortable with their feelings, ask yourself why. Wouldn't you let a child run and laugh and sing at the top of their lungs? Then let them have their other experiences at full blast, too. They need to know what happens as feelings bubble up in them, and they need to know the color of each feeling and its tones too, every intensity. It is a part of the literacy you can help them achieve.

Rewrite the Code: A mother can create safe spaces and resilience for her children to have the full experience of life, and it is further worthwhile for her to do it along with them.

Expecting mothers to do it all is expecting the impossible, and it is taking its toll on primary caregivers. We saw it all come crashing down during the pandemic, when primary caregivers were even more isolated, without school or activities to support the children. The burnout was real, and we are still recovering and healing. Unfortunately, with everything going back to business as usual, we can pretend again that our need for workability and understanding of the demands placed on us are untenable over the long term.

While I have mentioned this earlier, it bears repeating here that the United States is the only developed country that does not require paid leave for all mothers. Individual companies are changing their policies to encompass more flexibility and extended leave for new parents, which is great if you work at one of those companies. Sadly, most women, especially in marginalized communities, are not offered this benefit. We are crumbling under the weight of this pressure to be stretched so thin. I fear the consequences if we don't advocate in earnest for change.

Rewrite the Code: A woman is more than capable of providing high-quality care to both her job and her children when given adequate support and flexibility.

These seven examples by no means compile an exhaustive list of Mother Codes, and there is a plethora of nuances to each of them, but I have given you plenty to chew on and provide a thoughtful, personal inquiry. Don't let that stop you from continuing to build the list with ones that carry significant meaning to you and your family.

Albert Einstein aptly stated, "Blind obedience to authority is the greatest enemy of the truth." Your personal truth that casts your rainbow of color is something you are cultivating throughout this exploration of self-aware mothering, and it is priceless. It is just as true to say: Blind obedience to the Mother Codes is the greatest enemy to your transformative experience in motherhood.

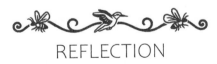

REFLECTION

Shine your light on the seven Mother Codes shared in this chapter. What was revealed for you?

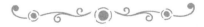

The splendor and glory of a rainbow do not exist in a vacuum or by magic. It appears in the presence of a rainstorm where sunlight and rain-filled clouds dance together in the sky. The darker the storm that coexists in the same space of the sky, the brighter and deeper the colors appear. We usually ignore the storm, but both are beautiful in their own right.

Codes are powerful. There is truth in the codes, yet the pure truth that lies within has been distorted. Caring for our children is a priority, but so is caring for mom. Of course, having irresponsible emotions around our children is harmful, but building strong social-emotional intelligence skills creates a family atmosphere where it is safe for everyone to be themselves fully.

I hope that by naming the most pervasive codes operating in our culture and offering ways for you to identify them personally as they manifested in your life, your awareness of how they have impacted you is growing. This is an interactive process, and you will continue to peel away the many layers of codes, like paint on a wall, that have accumulated year after year, generation after generation, of families, cultures, and systems. As you identify the codes within each layer, your awareness will expand and will lead to more self-awarenesses and more healing. With each new awareness, a facet of your prism comes online and becomes available for light to come through.

You become brighter and more accessible, and while you may be shy at first, to be this exposed, you will start to embrace it. And that is an awesome sight to behold!

Chapter 5

Rewrite YOUR Mother Code

Welcome to the midpoint of our journey together! I am delighted to see you here! You have accepted the invitation and opened the door to join women everywhere who are rewriting their Mother Codes and tuning into the frequency of the Cosmic Codes. I celebrate you! It is a big and beautiful step, and my heart is leaping for joy!

Rewriting the Mother Code is an awakening process. This compass will guide you out of a maze of propaganda and illusion that has all but convinced you that being a mother is about everything except for your power and your development. This old code has convinced you to push your needs down for others; be a servant to your partner and children; put away all other ambitions (or meet them and feel guilty); and live scripts written by your families and culture. Getting from this point to authentic personal development for yourself and leading growth for your whole family is not an easy task, but every small step you take will be rewarded with an increased sense of purpose.

Rewriting the Mother Code is not a one-and-done proposition.

If you truly dedicate yourself to this practice, you will spend the rest of your life growing into a new matricentric worldview. It will never end—and this is a good thing because it will also be endlessly nourishing and a source of hope and strength.

You have started a journey of creation, and you are now entering the garden in which you will cultivate yourself and your family differently. The time has come for you to write YOUR Mother Code. You have bravely lifted the veil and opened your eyes to an unvarnished world of motherhood as we are living it in our current culture. You have gathered data on what you like and don't like about how you have been programmed to view the mothering world you have entered or are about to enter. Without even knowing it, you have begun to open yourself to the Cosmic Codes. The time has come to pull all this treasure together into a statement that will act as your pillar, guide, rudder, and beacon, in and through your mothering exploration. I am honored to be on this path with you as you claim your dream. I will hold your hand as you touch your heart and reach into your soul for words to express the essence of your mothering experience.

Getting in the right mindset as you create will enhance your experience. Think of it almost as you would preparing mentally and physically for a trip or excursion into a new place. Or think of a little juicer example of setting up the space for foreplay and beyond in the bedroom. Either way, I want you to be as fully conscious and aware as possible! This endeavor calls you to set the worries and concerns of the moment aside and put your complete attention and presence into the experience.

While the Mother Code you birth and claim as your own will be a linear collection of words, they are words chosen by you to reflect your dreams and what matters to you at your deepest core level. It is a living and breathing entity—if you let it be. Your creation will be a mixture of elements pulled *out* from the depths of you and pulled *in* from the cosmos that together combine and alchemize. Words have power. Writing and speaking these words bring them to life and they are imbued with the energy you have given them.

To be clear, your Mother Code isn't a jumble of platitudes. It isn't what you **think** your mothering journey *should* be. It isn't superficial. It doesn't sound good but has hollow meaning to you. It also isn't a meek report that fosters a survival mentality. Maya Angelou's vision for us is to "not merely to survive, but to thrive; and to do so with some passion, some compassion, some humor, and some style." These words are your permission slip to dream big and be audacious in your desiring.

This is a space where creation takes place. You can feel the embodied pleasure of engaging with your full VOICE—both your inside voice and your outside voice—to bring to life your Mother Code!

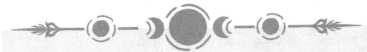

MOON RITUAL

Grandmother Moon sings to the seas who respond with the ebb and flow of the tides. She uses her energy to connect all of her daughters and granddaughters in the unifying experience of monthly bleeding. We respond to her call to shed what no longer brings life and open a space for creation to take place.

As evening falls and the moon begins to rise, find a peaceful spot or imagine one in your mind's eye where you can connect with its gentle glow. Reflect quietly on all that has happened in your day, acknowledging both the challenges and the moments of joy. Thank yourself for all that you've done, embracing the nurturing role you play.

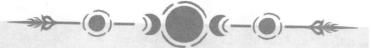

Gaze at the moon, or hold its image in your mind, and softly say, "As the moon renews itself, so do I. I release what no longer serves me."

Feel the calming light of the moon enveloping you, bringing peace and serenity, knowing that each night brings a new beginning.

A New Language

Transcending messages encoded from our lineage, from our culture, from science, philosophy, or religion are the codes comprising the truths of the universe. I call them Cosmic Codes. Residing within you at this very moment is the wisdom of the infinite. Pause and take that in. I mean *really* take that in. The stuff prophets, saints, and sages are made of isn't some anomaly bestowed on a chosen few—that stuff is in all of us. That may seem blasphemous, and at various points in history, a person could be killed for uttering such words. But now we can recognize that gut clench for what it is—a code imposed on us to limit our power and to keep us under control.

There is an essential distinction between the Cosmic Codes, the personal codes you developed as a child, and the cultural codes that surround us. These other two categories are human-made adaptations of the Mother Code. Personal and cultural codes are designed to advance the priorities of society, even if it is at your expense. Cosmic Codes speak directly to the nature of existence. They are unerring because they are the point of reference from which all other codes are derived. In the case of the Cosmic Codes, we are learning to tap into them, not change them. With childhood and cultural codes, we are taking control of what others have crafted and imposed on us.

The Cosmic Codes you will access as you rewrite your Mother Code go beyond limited definitions that restrict possibilities. Instead, it's about finding that spark inside of you that speaks to a wider, broader, and deeper consciousness. Feelings, images, and ideas will emerge that can be generally categorized (religion, science, philosophy etc.), but don't let that be your starting point. A "religion" category that then lists ideas of mother will produce a different concept than what emerges from your contemplation of a cosmic mother or motherhood without limits. The same goes with ideas of the mother images you saw around you in your family and culture and all the others. I shudder and tears come to my eyes when I think of limiting the possibilities of motherhood when restricted to the limits of science and biology.

Once you get into it, you might reasonably ask, if the Mother Code that society imprints upon us is harmful, then why shouldn't I be angry about it? And why shouldn't I act on that anger? Why shouldn't I want to destroy it?

This is definitely worth taking a moment to discuss.

Much of the Mother Code in our society reflects recent ideas, but no culture can erase the much deeper connection we have to mothers and mothering. I want you to see where the Mother Code framework under which you are operating now is limiting your development. But I don't want you to have the impression that we're throwing out the entire system and replacing it with a new one like it's a lightbulb or an air filter.

While the modern Mother Code does create conflict between mothering (as it defines it) and personal development, that doesn't mean being a mother today inherently imposes that conflict upon you. We must redefine what it means to be a mother in 21st century America. It's more about imposing balance than throwing bombs—literally or figuratively.

A lot of the cultural critique that is popular these days will tell you that "everything is wrong with X" or "you've been doing Y wrong this whole time." I believe these sweeping statements have less to do with some absolute flaw in humanity which has only just been uncovered and more to do with a collective yearning for a firmer foundation. I relate to this! The world can feel out of balance, with the ground under us shifting all the time, but the impulse to think in absolutes or to destroy rather than reshape is adding fuel to the fire. It is a very agentic, very aggressive framework that looks for things to smash.

To describe this phenomenon in the broadest terms, our society is out of balance, and at its core, that imbalance is about excessively masculine cultural programming. All our focus on materialism and winning and war is connected to a worldview that underestimates the power of the feminine to be a part of effective, lasting change. It's not even about whether feminine energy is better than masculine energy or women over men. It's about including feminine energy in how society shapes the world. Even when we glean some insight about the state of things, as we begin to reach for solutions, it is tempting to throw the baby out with the bathwater. But that's something mothers simply don't do.

Get angry about the limits that have been unjustly set on you as a mother if that is what you're feeling. You have a right to be angry! I am! I am furious that women have been put under a spell and believe it is acceptable and even noble to shrink ourselves. I am enraged that we are trained to separate ourselves from—and worse, fear—our own bodies. We are inundated with techno-medical advances that have stripped us of our embodied experience, most notably in conception, birth and new motherhood. So, yeah, I am angry.

We all should feel some righteous indignation at how we have been mistreated as mothers. But then we should take that energy and turn it into a productive purpose—rebalancing the society that gave rise to those injustices. And the place to start is within yourself.

Don't underestimate the power of your Mother Code and that of the other mothers taking this path of reinvention and personal development. Remember that at some point in time, huge systems like capitalism and science were the ideas of a few people, and over time, they began to gain influence one person at a time. You are a pioneer in the remaking of your own family and the human family. This is a powerful legacy that goes beyond the personal injury we have suffered, even as it honors our trauma and pain, to influence the future deeply and powerfully.

When you consider that the work we are doing to reawaken the Cosmic Codes within us will immediately begin to shape future generations, that influence quickly becomes exponential. Raising your children within the framework of your Mother Code means they will do the same, to some degree—it will be written in their identity the way your current Mother Code is written in yours. And their children will inherit that same framework. And so on. The nourishing, healing space you are creating for yourself will double, and then quadruple, and then multiply eightfold, and so on.

And just as we know and understand that everyone mothers and that mothering can mean many things to many people, so, too, the children of our ideas are our children in their own right. Influencing anyone to engage in this work means you have fostered a new seed of change in a new arc of influence. Your influence in this endeavor can ripple out into the world sooner and will have more impact than you may imagine.

So, I repeat, we should be angry at the injustice we have suffered, but we should not let that anger define us or live in us. Instead, the power we will use to erase the source of that injury should be what we pass down rather than bestowing fear, anger, hurt, and a hunger for revenge that keeps that suffering alive and spreading out of control. I hope that we become a force that reduces suffering, and grows into a chorus of hope rather than an army of hate.

Oh, the places we can go when we step out of the limiting paradigms and the structures the Mother Codes bind us to. What a glorious experience mothering can be! It is so much more than any of us realize. I know that I am bringing forth something I don't even understand. I am pregnant with an idea, a concept that lives deep in me and has for all women through time. I am reawakening it for myself and giving it form so we can all have access to it and help it grow.

We are manifesting a spec of what is possible for our lived human experience. I want to have us touch that which lies beyond our ordinary known reality. I want us to be in the explosive big bang of conception, the vast expansion of pregnancy, and the glorious miracle of birth in all manners and manifestations—a baby being just one of them.

What fusion of desires, what wondrous worlds of possibility can we behold? Let's go on a ride, the ride of our lives with the top down and wind blowing across our cheeks. Yes, it's messy. Yes, it's chaotic. Yes, it's ecstatic. Let's discover what love really is and what living a life of love can feel like. Let's change the makeup of our brains and leap to the next level of human existence. Let's feel all the lifetimes that have come before us. Let's taste the beauty of love and light and dark and mysterious.

Sure, there is some work to be done to get there, but when has that stopped us? Will we relent when the path becomes hard or dangerous? When we orient ourselves to love and resonate with the high vibrations of our combined voices, it is so much easier than we are led to believe. If you choose to mute your VOICE, you will be subjected to the voice of the prevailing culture. If you choose to activate your VOICE, you will open access to the voice of the Universe and the Cosmic Codes that reside there. So, I ask you, which do you choose?

Use Your VOICE for Creation

Surrendering into and opening your VOICE box is where the magic happens. Allowing access to your full range of voices, with emotional connection, will provide a conduit of expression and pleasure that is right and true for you.

V—Vision
O—Own
I—Intuition
C—Culture
E—Engage

Dropping into the space of *vision* loosens the reins of the linear and takes you into the vastness of the present moment. Seeing clearly for yourself will come from the mystical intuition and insight of your third eye. Visioning is a sensual experience grounded in sight, smell, taste, hearing, and touch.

You alone will *own* this space. Using words that are available to all and while familiar to you will become personal as you claim ownership of them. Your intention will infuse your words with power and potential that transcends temporal limitations.

Your *intuition* resides deep inside of you and is accessible the moment you call upon it. While direct and clear, it is also beyond reasoning. You are born with this knowing. And while words will fail to encompass the depth and breadth of your heartfelt passion, they will stand in as placeholders and portals of access to what lies beyond.

The creation of a personal *culture* is limitless in possibilities. Your words reflect your inherent belonging to the community of humankind in parallel with your unique fingerprint of existence. An authentic reflection of the alchemy that is you automatically raises the vibration of the community you surround yourself with. You will attract and build on each other's creative momentum.

Engaging with the life force and energy accessible in each word sparks creation. Words such as trust, vitality, play, truth, beauty, and love dance with rhythmic, pulsing, and ecstatic beats. When you engage in the creation and lived experience of your Mother Code, you will soar to new heights and be held in the arms of love and compassion.

Your Mother Code is something that delights you, and reflects your most authentic self that stems from your values, principles, *and* your wounds. It has the power to move you to tears and send waves of orgasmic joy through your whole body when you read it.

Mother Code 101—Four steps to crafting your Mother Code

Who doesn't love a good step-by-step process?! It's like following a recipe where you don't have to think or analyze, you just do the steps. You will gather ingredients, mix them, taste test, adjust, and voila, you have your Mother Code! I also like to think of following a recipe as the masculine system of a list and linear directions in service of the feminine creation that uses the process as a jumping-off point and more of a guideline than a rigid list of must-dos.

If cooking isn't your thing, think of how sheet music is essential to performance, but it takes the living presence and interpretation of that musical notation to make it sing (literally). Or how poems transform when read. The way we capture the spirit of a created thing lets it endure, but in many cases, for life to be breathed into it once again, it must be reanimated with the soul and passion of full presence in the moment.

The more attention you put into the physical and emotional space you are in, the more you will infuse your process with the love and care it warrants and ultimately is felt in your words. Clear your desk or space of clutter. If you have smudge or palo santo, light it and cleanse yourself and your space of any stagnant, destructive, or harmful energy and any blocks in the way. Light a candle and put on music that is uplifting and supportive of creative flow. This isn't a homework assignment on which you will be graded. Quite the opposite—it is a ceremony and rite of passage. You are marking a turning point in your life. Nothing will be the same going forward. You will see the world with new eyes and interact with new insights.

Step 1: Gather the essential elements.
Gathering the ingredients for your Mother Code statement is the place to start. The good news is you already have them all in your cupboard. Your Cosmic Codes have no expiration date and last a lifetime and beyond! They may have gotten hidden behind items put there by your mother, or you bought them because Instagram thought you should have them. Move those aside and there you will find many yummy and nourishing ingredients. Items such as the ones you found when you explored what you liked about the mothering you received. Harvest the work you did on family patterns and cull out positive themes you want to carry forward.

Values and principles
Values and principles are prime elements available to you. They come in many varieties, so let's select ones that light you up, nourish you, and call you to your highest. There is no scarcity here and I want you to feel like you can have them all if you so choose. Values and principles are closely related ideas, but they serve different roles in guiding thoughtful behavior and decision-making.

Values are the deep-rooted beliefs and ideals that form the bedrock of who you are. They're the inner compass guiding our actions, shaping our decisions, and defining what we hold dear in life. Think of them as the guiding stars in the constellation of your existence. These values are deeply personal and influenced by our experiences, upbringing, and culture. Integrity, honesty, compassion, respect, and responsibility are examples of these guiding lights illuminating your path through life.

Principles are the actionable guidelines we derive from these values. They're the practical rules that govern our behavior and decision-making in specific situations. While values provide the overarching framework, principles offer the nitty-gritty details, telling us how to act and what standards to uphold in various circumstances. Derived from our values, principles are more objective and universal, applicable across different contexts. For example, honesty translates into the principle of truthfulness, while fairness becomes the principle of justice.

To summarize, values are the ideals we hold dear; principles are the roadmaps guiding us on our journey. They're flexible enough to adapt to different situations yet grounded in the solid foundation of our values. Principles help us navigate the complexities of life, providing clarity and direction when faced with difficult choices. They're like the tools in our tool kit, ready to be wielded as we navigate the twists and turns of our individual paths. Values are the core of who we are, while principles are the actionable guidelines derived from those values, helping us live in alignment with what we hold dear. Together, they form the framework on which we build our lives, guiding us toward fulfillment, purpose, and authenticity.

Start with *values*, and make a list of as many values as you can name. See what you come up with at a first pass of heart-storming. I also share some examples here that may inspire and resonate with you.

What do you notice when you read these lists? How do you feel? Say them out loud, in order, and see where they land in your body. If the first group feels like they have a different resonance from the second group, you are picking up on the distinction between feminine (Yin) and masculine (Yang) values. No worries if you didn't feel a difference. I purposely grouped them this way so you can start making these distinctions in your life and in creating your Mother Code. They are equal in value but have a different energy and vibration. If you gravitate more toward one group than the other, that is rich data. It can both inform you where you orient and open possibilities to deepen those for yourself or expand into values from the other group. I suggest having a balance of both in your Mother Code statement.

Yin values		Yang values	
Nurturance	Providing care, support, and emotional warmth to others	Protection	Demonstrating physical, emotional, and mental resilience and fortitude
Cooperation	Emphasizing collaboration, consensus-building, and relationship-building	Competitiveness	Striving for achievement, success, and excellence in one's endeavors
Intuition	Trusting one's inner wisdom, gut feelings, and emotional insights	Logic	Emphasizing rationality, critical thinking, and problem-solving skills
Sensitivity	Being attuned to the emotions and needs of oneself and others	Assertiveness	Expressing oneself confidently, setting boundaries, and advocating for one's needs
Community	Prioritizing the well-being and interconnectedness of groups, families, and communities	Autonomy	Valuing self-reliance, personal freedom, and self-sufficiency
Fairness	Treating all people equally; giving everyone a chance to have their say; following a set of rules that everyone must abide by	Justice	Upholding fairness, equality, and moral principles in interactions and decisions
Flexibility	Adapting to change, embracing ambiguity, and finding creative solutions	Dominance	Control over one's environment and everyone and everything within it; expanding one's territory or sphere of influence
Connection	Valuing close relationships, intimacy, and emotional bonding	Bonding	Connections form through shared struggle and shared victory; tribal orientation
Harmony	Seeking peace, balance, and cooperation in relationships and environments	Victory	Prevailing over enemies; dominating opposition

Values Related to the Mother Code

Now that you have made a nice broad list, I want you to home in on no more than seven that most make your heart sing and resonate with you. Despite how many you are starting with, let all but seven fall through the strainer. Don't throw them away, just put them to the side as they are still valuable as a reference. You will take the list of your top seven with you as you create your Mother Code statement.

Great work! Now that you have the hang of this process, let's do the same with *principles*. First brainstorm any that come to mind immediately. Look over these groupings and see if there are any you want to add to your list. Choose your top seven principles to have as potential contributions to your Mother Code.

As you reflect on these facets of yourself, you are taking possession of who you are, literally explaining yourself to yourself. The person who comes into focus as you assemble the words that most resonate for you through this exercise may surprise you a little, or you may find yourself face-to-face with an old friend. No matter how you are becoming, you are leaning into a version of your Mother Code that is altogether yours in a way that has not been before, and you are connecting with the self within you that is beyond the rules of one family, one set of cultural norms, one society.

You are channeling what Zen Buddhist and instructor Dainin Katagiri calls The Light that Shines through Infinity—your cosmic self.

Crowdsource Codes

Noticing people you admire living in ways that inspire you can also inform your Mother Code. Do you have role models or people you see aspiring to live values and principles you resonate with? Who do you look up to? Who are your heroines? Maybe you haven't thought about this before. If so, start noticing how people around you operate and go about their days and nights and see what you resonate with in their way of being. You can also look to movies, shows, and books.

Yin values		Yang values
Nurturance	Providing care, support, and emotional warmth to others	Protection
Cooperation	Emphasizing collaboration, consensus-building, and relationship-building	Competitiveness
Intuition	Trusting one's inner wisdom, gut feelings, and emotional insights	Logic
Sensitivity	Being attuned to the emotions and needs of oneself and others	Assertiveness
Community	Prioritizing the well-being and interconnectedness of groups, families, and communities	Autonomy
Fairness	Treating all people equally; giving everyone a chance to have their say; following a set of rules that everyone must abide by	Justice
Flexibility	Adapting to change, embracing ambiguity, and finding creative solutions	Dominance
Connection	Valuing close relationships, intimacy, and emotional bonding	Bonding
Harmony	Seeking peace, balance, and cooperation in relationships and environments	Victory

	RMC principles	RMC statement of principle
Demonstrating physical, emotional, and mental resilience and fortitude	Strength	Using one's full strength, helping others to flourish while making safe space for each and all
Striving for achievement, success, and excellence in one's endeavors	Accomplishment	Successfully reaching outcomes through a balance of personal initiative and team effort
Emphasizing rationality, critical thinking, and problem-solving skills	Intelligence	Cultivating one's total intelligence to understand oneself, the people around you, the world, and the cosmos
Expressing oneself confidently, setting boundaries, and advocating for one's needs	Rapport	Communicating in a way which values indivudals and the group, ensuring each person is heard by and hear others
Valuing self-reliance, personal freedom, and self-sufficiency	Civitas	Organizing people within society—or the entirety of a society—to flourish as a collective while nurturing the leadership skills of individuals in areas that benefit themselves and others
Upholding fairness, equality, and moral principles in interactions and decisions	Empowerment	Providing people with the tools to be self-sufficient and also a benefit to the collective and overseeing everyone to ensure that the behavior of one person or group does not diminish the freedoms and rights of another person or group
Control over one's environment and everyone and everything within it; expanding one's territory or sphere of influence	Stewardship	Decision making which allows for the unexpected and original while safeguarding some degree of collective consensus
Connections form through shared struggle and shared victory; tribal orientation	Engagement	Forming groups based on affinity and need and allowing people to thrive within those groups in whichever ways are best for their development that do not harm or limit others
Prevailing over enemies; dominating opposition	Governance	Maintaining social order while holding space for a variety of ways to live within a society

Remarkably, when you begin to dig deep into the stories of famous women, you'll see many are known for their professional achievements and yet their notable approaches to mothering are all but erased. Marie Curie is a good example of this. She is famous for her work in radiation, but she has a much more textured life than the sound bites during Women's History Month suggest.

Marie had to raise her two daughters on her own following the death of her husband Pierre, who died in an accident. Dissatisfied with the education system in Paris, she homeschooled her children alongside other accomplished scientists in the city. Each scientist taught in their area of expertise, and the children seem to have thrived in that arrangement.[1] Irene Curie—later Joliot-Curie—followed in her mother's footsteps in terms of pursuing research on radioactivity and excelling in it. She received her own Nobel Prize in 1935.

History is full of examples of mothers who blazed their own trails and passed on their codes of independent thinking and living to their children. There are also women who have advocated for a more expansive view of motherhood and who have written their own codes but chose not to have children. They are as much a part of the story as anyone else. Lydia Maria Child, for example, is a woman who lived in New England in the 19th century and tirelessly fought for the rights of oppressed people, including enslaved people and women. She was a dedicated abolitionist and the breadwinner in her family, making a living through all sorts of writing. She published her first novel at 22 and is known for advocating for equality for women. In her book of advice for mothers, *The Mother's Book*, she observes that:

> "The great difficulty at the present day is that matrimony is made a subject of pride, vanity, or

---

1   You can read more about Marie Curie's mothering and her daughters at https://engines.egr.uh.edu/episode/3087.

expediency, whereas it ought to be a matter of free choice and honest preference. A woman educated with proper views on the subject could not be excessively troubled at not being married, when in fact she had never seen a person for whom she entertained particular affection; but one taught to regard it as a matter of pride, is inevitably wretched, discontented, and envious, under the prospect of being an old maid, though she regards no human being with anything like love."[2]

She also advised that sometimes, the needs of children should *not* come first. This is Mother Code 101! You can imagine how unpopular that view was when she published this book in 1831. Lydia's willingness to speak the truth in the face of limiting traditions—including the Mother Code—led to a great deal of hardship in her life, but she publicly declared that she had no regrets for speaking out for what's right.

And to be clear, these are not special women who lived grand, remarkable lives. They used their VOICE and particularly *owned* their lives and their experiences. It is incredible to make an impact in science so significant that you win a Nobel Prize. I contend that it is equally award-worthy to homeschool your children while you are doing it. The point is to see the lives of these women not as some unattainable ideal but as a beacon of what is possible.

Imagine Your Ideal Day as a Mother

I invite you to create a video in your mind that spans a full 24 hours, showing an ideal day in your life. You can do this as a meditation if you like. With your eyes closed, picture as many moments as you can from the time you wake up, through your whole day,

---

2 The full text of this fascinating book is archived at https://digital.library.upenn.edu/women/child/book/book.html.

bedtime, and then even through your sleep and dream time. Be as detailed as possible. How do you feel at any given moment? How do you handle challenges and upsets as they will inevitably come up? Imagine the ways you will take care of yourself throughout the day. Envision yourself living the values and principles in as many moments as you can. And don't worry if this doesn't come easy. It may be hard to imagine something you haven't lived yet.

I know for me, it was more comfortable to picture basically the same day with just a little improvement. Or imagining engaging in my unhealthy behaviors a little less. While this is the pathway that leads to your ideal, it helps to envision yourself already there and the many positive outcomes that emerge.

A word of warning—your brain will not like this exercise at all! It will try to shut this dreaming of possibilities right down because it does not like change. Resist the pull as best you can and continue to bring yourself back to the images of your ideal day. Being curious about your resistance may not sound immediately appealing, but that is where the growth happens. Choosing to orient to values and principles often invites a reckoning of where we have and have not been living them.

I had always considered myself a pretty honest person, but when I shined the light onto my prism, specifically on living the value of honesty and the principle of truthfulness, a lot came to the surface—and it wasn't pretty. Living lie-free sounded like a nice idea, but it turned out to be more like an alcoholic getting sober. A fearless inventory of all the ways I lied by omission, "softened" the truth, and even told bald-faced lies reflected a distorted image I had held of myself as honest. It was a relief and actually quite freeing to fess up to where and how much I wasn't telling the truth.

But I broke down when I tried to imagine living a 100% honest life in total alignment with my truth. It was a really beautiful image, but I feared that if I was that honest and that authentic, I not only wouldn't be liked but I would also be abandoned. This imagined fear wielded a lot of power and shut me down from even thinking about the possibility. It took some work to take the risk and let myself imagine how at peace I would feel and how powerful sharing my truth from a place of vision could be. Yes, some people did not like it, so it led to envisioning such a strong core sense of self I could weather these interactions and losses.

I hope you are seeing the power these words hold in our healing and transformation process. They are a beacon for us around which we can orient and journey into the depths of our being. Sometimes, it leads us into the shadow sides of ourselves and the more we can see this as a beautiful thing, the more power your Mother Code statement will have.

Step 2: Helpful guidelines before you combine elements.

Creative expression can sometimes feel like a lot of pressure, and that can make the process difficult. A blank page staring up at you has the power to paralyze even the most prolific writers! I know I have myriad avoidance and stalling tactics that slow down my creative process.

Have you ever felt like you have nothing to say or no imagination? You're not alone! But it is almost always the case that barriers are between us and the ideas inside of us, and nine times out of ten, we've put them there ourselves, which means we can remove them as well. The word *express* is an important aspect of creativity. It has its origins in the Latin *pressare*, to press. Expressing an idea is a matter of releasing something that already exists inside of you. If you run into difficulties doing this, consider whether you've blocked the flow the way rocks can dam up a stream.

For example, negative language makes it especially difficult to express a vision, and this is a main source of blockage when trying to get those ideas to flow. Avoid expressing ideas about yourself in the negative. Talking about what you can't do or won't do or haven't done does not get you closer to what you will do or what you are doing now. Pull those rocks out of the stream! Let it flow!

Thinking about the process is less useful than engaging in it. The best solution for a creative block is to create. Spending all your time trying to get in the right state of mind or wondering what you ought to express has almost no value when compared to actually creating. Streams do not think about flowing to flow. Movement is inherently a part of being a stream. Who you want to be is a part of who you are. You have this within you and need only get out of its way for it to start manifesting.

Our whole society overthinks everything and yet doesn't think clearly about very much at all. We depend on our analytical, conscious brain and ignore whole other elements of thought, including intuition, heart-led reasoning, and even the subconscious. Your Mother Code is a chance to move outside of that paradigm, which has not been nourishing to the world.

As you begin the process of creating your Mother Code, I want to remind you that mothers in all forms are the only authentic creators. Artists rearrange material in the world. Writers reorganize words that have been used repeatedly countless times. Mothers combine elements from disparate sources and create entire living beings from them—new cells, bones, blood, skin, brains are all created by the mother. It is the only real creation, and you are the author of this potentiality. A mother no more has to will a baby to grow within the womb than a river has to decide the course it will take. And your Mother Code, which is the best expression of you, is also within you, waiting to be expressed. Simply let it out.

When you get ready to start writing, here are a few suggestions. Take what is helpful and disregard the rest:

- Be creative with your format—writing, drawing, sculpting, poetry.

- Dream big! Let yourself be audacious in your wanting for yourself.

- Use positive language—our brain can't do a don't so stay in the affirmative.

- Harness the power of your senses—see it, hear it, taste it, smell it, touch it. Sensual language grounds you in the present moment.

- Keep going—even if what you are imagining for yourself feels impossible at this moment.

- Write from the present tense as if what you are writing has happened and you are describing it.

- Claim it fully without ambiguity. "I am..." is more powerful than "I will be..."

- Write in community with one or more other like-minded people. You are giving birth to a new you, after all!

Step 3: Combine ingredients.

Before you overthink it or make too big of a deal about it, write a first draft of your Mother Code. You have done the hard work, and now let your first pass float to the surface. I suggest setting a timer for no more than three minutes and let whatever flows from you come out. You can also speak it into a voice note for up to three minutes.

Whatever lands on the page is of value. It may feel just right from the start. Or you may notice you left out a key ingredient, so you add it in. If you wrote in bullet points, take another few minutes to turn them into sentences.

Size matters (but not how you think it does!). Being super detailed and painting a thorough picture will serve you well. I encourage you to do so if it pleases you, but it is not required.

Ultimately, you will want to create a one- to three-sentence distilled version you can hold in your mind and refer to easily. It won't have all the detail, but it will reflect the essence of it.

Feelings check—use your emotions to test and guide you until your Mother Code is just right. Think of *Goldie Locks and the Three Bears,* where she tastes the porridge, sits in the chairs, and lays down on the beds until she finds the ones that are "just right!"

Now, sit with what has come through for you. Let it marinate overnight or for some days, and then come back to it. How does it feel? Does it need any adjustments, or does it feel good as it is? If you want to deepen or play with it further you can review your lists, meditate on it, and make revisions accordingly. I encourage you to let your intuition guide you and have a sense of resonance that feels both pleasing as well as challenging to be your guide.

Remember, there is no right or wrong here and perfectionism will most assuredly kill the vibe. Find a balance of loving it and accepting it. In my experience, people generally get to something very close after one or two passes at it. When I coach someone through this, I may offer some language support to make sure it is written in the positive and you are claiming it fully. For example, I may tweak a statement from "I will be a woman who doesn't resist change" to "I am a woman who embraces change."

When you feel ready, say it out loud. Say it like you mean it! Use your voice and claim it fully as yours.

Step 4: Enjoy your creation!

Whether celebrating milestones and important events is part of your vision or not, it is time to minimally do a little happy dance or, even better, a full-out celebration. You have done it! You may have thought you were throwing a little something together, but you have done way more than that. You have given birth to your Mother Code. And that, my friend, is a big fu&*ing deal!

Whether you went super deep in your exploration and made the experience part of a personal growth and healing process, came to it from a rite of passage vantage point, or took a few notes and jotted something meaningful down for yourself, it is all valuable. What matters is that you made it yours. You chose your pathway, and you engaged in a creative process. I am moved, delighted, and so proud of you. And unless you send it to me (which I would love!), I won't even know what it says, but I promise you, I will feel it.

I am not the only one who will feel it. People close to you will wonder what is different about you. They won't be able to quite pinpoint it, so they may think it is something external like you got a haircut or something. And even bigger than that, you have affected the greater good and made a difference in the world, which is no small matter!

I want you to bask in the glory and wonder of your creation. Sure, it may even be imperfect and not quite at its fullness. It is in its infancy, and it needs to be fed, protected, and engaged with. And like with your children, it will teach you, and you will teach it. You are in this together through thick and thin.

It is also more than okay to feel protective and reserved about sharing it at first. It is a tender shoot that just popped out of its seed and has broken ground. The last thing you want is for it to be stomped on by a casual passerby. Be a mama bear protecting her young. And know that sometimes it's best to practice not having to explain yourself to people. You are who you have always been—only more!

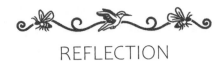

REFLECTION

As you celebrate your newly birthed Mother Code, continue to visualize what living it will bring you. Picture a scenario with someone where you felt challenged. Now, imagine how you could approach it if you bring in your Mother Code. What is one thing you would say or do differently?

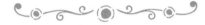

"I get it! I finally really get Rewrite the Mother Code! I just rewrote my birth story!" Lara exclaimed as she emerged from the water at the close of a breathwork activation I was guiding her through.

"Say more about that. And don't feel like you must make sense, just flow," I coaxed her, not wanting to get her too much in her head but still capture some of this profound moment in words.

Lara had shared with me, leading to our immersive experience, that the story she heard throughout her life was how difficult it was to give birth to her. Her mom was in labor for two days, and Lara wouldn't come. There was always a sense of blame and the belief that the labor was not only hard—Lara was hard. Being difficult was further exacerbated by being an inconsolable, colicky baby. This experience formed some of Lara's first coding and sense that she was too much or too big.

Knowing this about her birth story, I gave her the directive that at some point while she was in the womb-like atmosphere of the pool, she was to return to her birth. And return to her birth she did! I suspend logical and rational thinking when a client enters a wormhole back to a time in their past, as I believe we can not only heal cognitively but rewrite our past and create new memories.

Lara seized the opportunity and shared with me what she felt was her mother's resistance to letting go during the birth. She could feel her mother's fear and, in her effort not to cause her mother suffering, Lara held on as well. But at the moment her mother chose to surrender, Lara seized the opportunity to come forth. This was the truth of what happened, and by touching this space, Lara rewrote the negative attributes the previous story held for her.

It's a simple fact that many of us know nowhere near what we should about our bodies. The system has convinced us that bodies are a complicated business and should be left to professionals to poke, prod, assess, and generally discern. This is considered especially true for women and even more so regarding questions of fertility, pregnancy, and birth. Practices such as very expensive fertility regimes and freezing eggs (also very expensive) are a consequence of people who see the ability of a woman to conceive and give birth as a kind of mini-factory and focus on production over any holistic perspective.

This became very clear in my journey toward motherhood when I didn't have a period for months, and no medical explanation was forthcoming. As I shared in Chapter 3, it took a woman who was trained as a traditional MD, as well as Eastern and integrative medicine, to point out that I had made myself thin at an unhealthy level in the process of living my life and chasing my dream to have children. As I returned to something like a normal diet and weight, my period, too, returned. I tell this story to let women know that the messages imposed on us about what being healthy looks like are as flawed as the idea that the life-saving power of a C-section should become thoughtlessly routine.

I also want you to know that no misunderstanding about your body, no lack of information is a matter of shame. Let that be another badge of honor for you in the journey to rewriting your Mother Code. When you begin to more fully understand your body, you are taking possession of the legacy that is rightfully yours, and you should note every instance where you gained another piece of information that helped to form a fuller picture of who you are, inside and out.

When you first decided to read this book, you took an important step in your journey of self-discovery and self-determination. Setting your Mother Code down, in whatever way you have done that, is yet another milestone. Because we are deluged every day with so much information, it's easy to forget just how much power words have. But no matter how often words are used to sell things or lure you into clicking some button on your phone, that power is still within them, when used with intention and seriousness of purpose.

Mark this day on your calendar. Save the draft you have created of your statement of your Mother Code, even if you rewrite it (or resculpt it or resing it or ...). Because this expression has profound meaning, and in the story of you, what you have made today is of unique importance. Celebrate your creation and celebrate your vision of yourself as a mother that grows inside of you. You are stepping into a new perception of the world.

Along with all this seriousness, don't forget joy! Don't forget laughter! This is a time of tremendous freedom for you, a step on a path away from a long list of restrictions that should have never been placed on you. You are taking a deliberate turn toward freedom, toward the light of the sun. And while it may feel bittersweet and I encourage you to feel any sadness or fear or anger that arises, remember to be joyful—an expanded purpose is flowing into your life.

Chapter 6

Rising Into Motherhood

"I am not afraid of the pain!" Sanya proclaimed when she opened her eyes. It was the final breathwork session we would do together, just one month before the birth of her first child.

Having coached Sanya and her husband every step of the way from preparations for conception through the pregnancy itself, I knew what an epic statement this was for her. She had already engaged in deep and thoughtful personal work to identify and resolve so many family and cultural codes that it wasn't surprising she would reach this point, but it was profound.

Sanya started her pregnancy with a clear boundary—that she did not want me or anyone else to try and talk her into anything other than a medicalized hospital birth with a doctor. As challenging as this boundary was for me, I kept my mouth shut and honored her request as the one that was right for her. Mind you, I am careful never to push my agenda or opinion when I am coaching clients through pregnancy. But I always ask if they are interested in hearing my perspective and invite them into an inquiry that explores all options available. Through her own process, however,

Sanya had become curious about other possibilities. At her request, I opened the door, and she walked through it to the choices available to her, and from there, she determined her course of action.

At the start of her third trimester of pregnancy, after peeling away so many layers of family and cultural programming, she and her husband chose to switch to a midwife practice, create a birth plan that didn't include medication unless explicitly required, and hire a doula so she could labor at home for as long as possible. That is quite a 180-degree change in direction from where she started! They account for the shift to reorienting to the values and principles she and her husband had claimed in the vision they wrote for themselves and her rewritten Mother Codes. This vision included living to their full potential, healing generational trauma, freedom of emotional expression, and deepening their relationship with Allah.

"No, I am not afraid of the pain as I first thought," Sanya shared. "I am actually afraid of the aliveness and energy that will course through my body when I give birth. I am afraid I will not have the capacity to be with the intensity of this embodied experience. But then I imagined myself doing it and was not only capable of managing it, but I also inhabited it. I was a vessel containing aliveness and pure energy."

With this new vision overriding the old images from her past programming, Sanya felt ready for whatever course her birth would take.

I was invited to the birth, but her labor went so beautifully (most of which she did at home) that by the time I walked into her birthing room, what I witnessed was not a beleaguered woman but a beaming light. She was smiling ear to ear as if it had all been effortless, with her husband recounting the powerful and almost regal space she held through her labor and birth.

It is a great joy of my practice that I have been a companion to so many mothers and couples as they begin their journey into parenthood. And a divine motherhood glimmers inside every experience, just waiting to emerge and blossom from within. This same divinity resides within you, and as much as I am conveying to you all the complexities of the Mother Code, I want you to also understand this power of transformation is already a potentiality inside of you.

I've talked about the codes of motherhood and the many ways they show up in everyday life. I've shared how to recognize those codes and how you can become aware of instances of the code manifesting. I describe it as code because that's the best way to make the science of its neuro-conscious presence within you make sense while also pointing toward a method of transformation. I will continue to encourage and support you to find your own truths instead of the codes that hold you to oppressive standards because that is the central message of this book: You can build your vision of mothering that is as deeply a part of who you are as the alternatives have been.

These elements have been discussed in very practical ways because much of this work is just that—a practice. But the promise literally goes beyond the constraints of one's family, one's community, one's culture—and, ultimately, transcends even the limitations of the self.

Yes, this is holy work. Not so much in the religious sense, which has its own beauty and importance if it is a part of your life, but in a universal, nondogmatic way. I am calling attention to what is sacred in the mundane, in the daily practice. This is the profundity that lives in the margins and the simplest of spaces. I am aware that I am sharing some of my and others' peak experiences throughout this book, but how life is lived between such experiences in your day-to-day reality matters as much or more. Chasing spiritual experiences is not the game. Having transcended experiences, appreciating them, and then taking the messages and leaning into new behaviors, new thought patterns—that is where the magic lives.

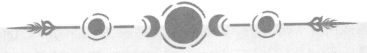

STAR RITUAL

Just as there are an infinite number of stars in the sky, every person's experience of mothering is unique and perfect for them. Does one star look across the vastness and seek to be like another? I cannot imagine this to be true.

Under the night sky or in your imagination, seek a star that draws your attention. Marvel at its distant light, imagining all the nights it has watched over. Hold a wish or intention in your heart, something for yourself, your child(ren), or your future. With a gentle whisper, send your wish to the star, believing it will carry your hopes into the vastness of the universe.

As you gaze at the stars, feel a deep connection to the infinite, knowing you are part of something greater. Conclude with a quiet affirmation: "As the stars shine brightly, so does my love and hope for the future."

Let this connection bring you awe and comfort.

Emerging from Behind the Veil

In our current culture, conception, pregnancy, and birth are becoming more and more shrouded in a veil of fear and scarcity. Our techno-medical culture preys on the vulnerability of a woman's desire and capacity to conceive and give birth. Women in their twenties are being advised that they better freeze their eggs and freeze them NOW! The urgency of this messaging is infusing fear they may lose their window of opportunity to conceive, and it can create a panic that feeds our primal scarcity mindset.

Our ability to probe inside a woman's ovaries and scientifically assess her egg count and viability for pregnancy is both wondrous and abhorrent. Wondrous because it is pretty cool to get a front row seat of our bodily processes. Abhorrent because we are programmed to put science and data on a pedestal and worship it as an all-knowing god. Talk about popping the balloon of wonder, mystery, and miracles! These are arenas where it is important for us to hold both perspectives and stay open to the values reflected in each paradigm.

Motherhood is one of the most vulnerable acts you will ever take part in because there is almost nothing you will care about as much or pour yourself so fully into as your child. This vulnerability and ambiguity about what the job entails can leave us wrought with guilt and feelings of not "enoughness." Studies show that many women in our culture feel unprepared for the journey of conception, pregnancy, birth, and especially new motherhood.[1] We have become isolated and no longer live in community with women of varying ages and experiences. Unless you work in a field where you are exposed to birth and new motherhood or grew up in a family where you were called to assist, it is an experience we only read about or see images of in movies and on social media.[2] Since the data reflecting the full expanse of possibilities is almost unavailable and favors options that perpetuate patriarchal ideals, it is incumbent on us to seek them out.

I remember when I was newly pregnant, and we were deciding between a midwife practice in a hospital or a home birth. At the

1   Here is a sample of the scholarship addressing this important issue: Leifer, Myra. *Psychological Effects of Motherhood: A Study of First Pregnancy*. New York, Praeger Publishers, 1980, esp. p. 20: "Most women began their pregnancy with little knowledge of what would occur."; Sciberras, Danica. *Pregnant women's expectations for the early postpartum period after their first childbirth*. BS thesis. University of Malta, 2022: "Many women perceive the early postpartum as a somewhat unknown and, to a certain extent, unknowable period for which they were largely ill equipped."

2   For one view on the impact of media representations of birth, see Cummins, Molly Wiant. "Miracles and home births: the importance of media representations of birth." *Critical Studies in Media Communication* 37.1 (2020): 85-96.

hospital, we were shown the facility and had the chance to meet with one of the midwives who told us what we could expect should we choose to give birth there. What I remember most from that visit was being told that if my pregnancy extended two weeks beyond my due date, they would induce me. I asked if there was any wiggle room with that if my and the baby's conditions were in good order. The response was, "No, that is our policy and under no circumstances will we diverge from it." I knew right then that the inflexible CYA (cover your ass) attitude of a hospital was a big red flag for me.

When we visited Chicago Community Midwives, a home birth practice that sadly no longer exists (because we are systematically making it impossible to practice midwifery outside a hospital setting in our country[3]), it was like being in someone's living room. It was the first floor of the residence of one of the midwives. While my husband and I waited to meet with one of the midwives, we were invited to look at the photo albums on the coffee table.

These albums turned out to be page after page of images of women giving birth in their homes. While looking at these images, I realized just how far removed I was from the real experience of birth. This was breaking rules and beliefs I didn't know I had. Beliefs such as birth being a private matter you don't share in a public photo album. I was both shocked and relieved, shocked by the in-my-face reality of the experience and relieved that it wasn't being hidden from me. I found it ironic that I felt less safe in the place that offered strict guidelines and medical technology at the ready than I did in the living room of this community of midwives. I was uncomfortable in both places, but the main differentiator was around agency with my body and choices.

Where did the longing for a birth experience free from the

---

3 In Chicago, where I raised my children, local media has done some reporting on this issue. See https://www.wbez.org/stories/midwives-fight-to-stay-at-chicago-area-hospitals/15b6c501-11d0-4ec6-9bc2-0c67f33badb1. For a national perspective, see https://www.commonwealthfund.org/publications/issue-briefs/2023/may/expanding-role-midwives-address-maternal-health-crisis.

constraints of modern technology come from in me? Rather than assume it was happenstance, I choose to believe that just because I am programmed with Mother Codes by my current family and culture in some disempowering ways, it doesn't mean I have lost the ancient wisdom that gives rise to a hunger for an embodied experience. That programming is in there too! I find this hopeful. Even though the universal wisdom of the ages may be in the far reaches of our conscious awareness, it is there patiently waiting for us to bring it back online.

Motherhood, when viewed as a person-centered, divine experience, offers opportunities for profound healing and transformation. This perspective coincides with conventional mystical practices, suggesting that experiences like pain, breath, sleep deprivation, and sexuality inherent in motherhood could lead to altered states.

Imagine breaking away from the patriarchal notion that the pain of childbirth was a punishment from God and instead reclaiming birth pain as the roller coaster we choose to ride with eyes wide open and hands up in the air, screaming in both terror and exhilaration. What if we viewed the nonlinear, unfocused experience of sleep deprivation in the first weeks and months of new motherhood as a built-in way to soften the edges in a dreamy state and render ourselves incapable of doing much else than being with our baby. These suggestions may sound outrageous, inconceivable, or even a little naughty, but I have firsthand experience both with myself and the women I coach that they are plausible.

Birth is an experience that is unique to people who have a uterus and can conceive, grow a baby inside their womb, and give birth.[4] When we say we are creative, when we say an artist creates a painting or sculpture, our original point of reference, the only

---

4 There are other, powerful experiences that are part of the birth of a child, and technology provides more and more options outside of this traditional experience. We can embrace all of those other happenings and the growth they bring without negating or mitigating the absolutely unique experience of a traditional birth cycle. In fact, without acknowledgement of the sacrality of the baseline event, all other, related events are cheapened.

truly original act on the planet, is to conceive and birth a living being. Consider how unique the knowledge and insight gained from that experience is.

In all meaningful creation, there is an element of courageous exploration. This is a safe place to explore, think, and say the unsayable—nothing is taboo as you create the mothering journey truly of your making. Given the audacious complexity of blazing your pathway toward a self-directed experience of mothering, I want to underline that this is a game of raising awareness, using your intuition, and making choices. Not just once but repeatedly. It's healthy to be curious and even suspicious at times of how the processes and norms surrounding motherhood came to be what they are.

This isn't about questioning everything or being paranoid that the world is out to get us. It is more about being open and willing to question some common thinking, such as, "This is how women in my family have always done it, so it must be good for me." Or "If the majority of the U.S. population gives birth in a hospital, it must be the safest way." The first clue as to when to consider questioning a current practice is if you have even the slightest gut clench or spark of wondering if there are also other ways to go about this endeavor.

Noticing Doubts

I am fond of religious iconography. It's no doubt a result, in part, of my Catholic upbringing, a religion that is chock full of paintings, statues, stained glass, and all sorts of other physical representations of the spiritual path. The early church did not have social media, so it put the pictures on the windows! It is no surprise to me then that I've had powerful moments in the presence of religious icons. I know more than one mother who has also had strong emotional moments while saying the rosary or praying in front of an image of a saint. That may not be your thing, but however you practice your faith or connect to the spiritual world, the settings in which you have felt any strong emotion are just as significant as my experience among the broken statues of Buddha and by the shrine to the Virgin Mary.

We often bury our feelings about spiritual matters, especially now when unbelief seems so popular and religion is derided as unsophisticated. Forget all that. When you reflect on your own life, you'll find that your moments of faith and doubt and fear and hope are all there, and those are powerful moments you should hold on to. No doubt some of those moments concerned your family or your children or your desire to have children. Hold onto those. They are an important part of the story of your Mother Code.

The stories of everyone around you whose experiences intersect with your mothering story are a part of your code—and can be a part of rewriting it. Long before I was a mother, I watched my grandparents model what a loving couple looked like and saw how that love spilled over into how they treated us. Those positive memories are a counterweight to the many challenging examples from my childhood, and all of it is a cumulative library of modeled behaviors (and my interactions with them).

We capture our memories and record our dreams differently. Whatever form you use can be a physical manifestation of those memories, whether it's journal entries, collage, audio recordings—any of it can be a part of your process of Rewriting the Mother Code.

But absences are also stories. When Rich and I decided not to share the news about my pregnancy for a while, there was a whole series of reasons behind it. I think, above all, we wanted to be firm in our understanding of what having a child would be like for us before people started telling us what it would be like. I was especially wary of the many horror stories that women will trot out about their own pregnancies and the effect they had on their body. So, we just didn't talk about it and instead did our own preparation. That choice to not act, to remain quiet, is an important part of my story and is built into my rewritten Mother Code. Written into my new code is the decision to say yes and no as I see fit, to not be pressured into other people's ideas about how pregnancy should happen. What you choose not to do is part of your story as well.

If the path to rewriting your Mother Code ever starts to feel like it's complicated to achieve, I am here to tell you it is not. Any doubts or reluctance are part of the spell we are under to keep us from tapping into our maternal power. When you begin to recognize these as limiting thoughts, and you catch one in action, take a beat and take stock of what you may have overlooked in your work. Consider, for example, my comments about how I reacted when I first read *What to Expect When You're Expecting*. (And let me say once again that I still found value in that book but also realized I needed other books to fill in gaps.)

I bought a book, I read some of it, I reacted to it, and I sought what I needed. That's a significant part of my story, no matter how basic the steps seem to be. Simply figuring out what's a good fit for you and what isn't is part of your process. Don't forget that an aggregate effect works especially well if you are aware you are rewriting your Code in the moment but also as you reflect on the choices you make and experiences you have which are related to your personal development. The key is to perceive them as such, as part of the process of creating your Code.

Noticing Regrets

Burying regrets of the choices we made is one of those internal reactions to painful emotions. It can become so routine within many of us that it acts like a reflex. The memory emerges, a flash of pain stabs us, and we shove it back down quickly. Regret is not your enemy! Let it fully unfold. What do you regret? Why do you regret it? Do you always feel that way, or is it just now, and if so, why now? When I laid bare my regrets at the broken Buddha temple on the Mekong River in Laos, it was anything but a pity party or beat-up session. Sharing my regrets about some of my mothering choices with raw vulnerability was the opening that let cosmic compassion flow into me.

Regrets are inevitable because we are all here for a short time, and we can't choose everything we want to do. You can't *have* children and also *not have* children. But I encourage you to have moments of acknowledging the loss of the other choice. Let the feelings happen, and let it pass. It is a central part of our development that we can face the human condition without fear. When I became pregnant for the second time, I hoped it would be another girl—and it was! It was not until I was facilitating a retreat with mothers and sons that I let myself feel the loss of this experience. While observing the unique dynamics and energy of boys, it suddenly struck me I would never have *that* experience. I opened myself to the sadness connected to this loss.

The more you embrace the experience of your loss and regrets, the more you develop as a person, and facing those regrets is a part of building the life—and the Mother Code—that you envision for yourself.

Sounding the Cosmic Call

Using the VOICE framework calls us to expand our *awareness* around all conventional knowledge related to parenting and mothering specifically. You will hear me say often throughout this book that awareness is the catalyst for Rewriting the Mother Code. It is our willingness to expand our field of vision as we look both inward, to become more self-aware, and outward, to explore possibilities.

Conscious awareness is a gift to be honored. This happening can take us from the mundane routine of life into the place of miracles. We have this incredible power to tap into the ever-present place of awareness. *Awareness is.* Pause for a moment and let that sink in. Awareness is always around you. Awareness hasn't evolved; it is just so. But we are evolving to be present to its invitation; to know that within us is the choice to take any act, any observation, any interaction and choose to be in awe and wonder. To be with awareness is to be in communion with that which is.

Birth is a wonder. Birth is a miracle. When we hold this, it is impossible not to see what is and is not in alignment with this truth. Our choices dictate whether we will either honor or dishonor this miracle. We can harness the full capacity of our brains where both logical and intuitive thinking reside, neither of which has more power or value than the other. The creation that comes from that space is a miracle of its own. Think of the brain as a womb of creation where different kinds of thinking interplay and connect and create our actions.

Splitting our brain into two equal halves with explicitly distinct jobs is simplistic and rarely honors the complexity and nuance of this magnificent human organ. With that caveat in mind, neuroscience research shows that *generally* our left brain keeps the lens we look through narrow and linear.[5] From an evolutionary perspective, narrow focus can be a good thing. For example, when the hunter (often but not always male) needed to have a long-range, narrow focus, tuning out their surroundings to stalk and kill the animal that would provide resources to the family or tribe, it was beneficial. The laser-focus part of the brain that tunes everything else out became highly developed for survival purposes. Whether men or women participated in hunts, it was always the left side of the brain that honed the hunter skill—a skill more highly valued in our current culture.

The gatherer needed a broader perspective and developed not only peripheral vision and heightened awareness of the sounds and activity around them, but also discernment in identifying and distinguishing nutritious and medicinal plants from poisonous ones. This provided the ability to gather more effectively, and the heightened awareness strengthened our radar to keep an eye on

---

5   A very readable breakdown of left brain and right brain characteristics can be found at https://www.verywellmind.com/left-brain-vs-right-brain-2795005.

the children. Contrary to popular belief that the hunter did the *important* job, it was mainly the women who, through their gathering, contributed 80% of the food and medicinal herbs needed for the tribe or family to survive. Just saying!

The legacy of that ancient pattern lives in the different ways in which male and female brains have evolved. Scientific analysis of the brain activity of men and women shows we will solve the same problem in two very different ways: The man activates a narrow part of the brain in a situation where a woman uses several areas of the brain to reach the same solution.[6] And this complex reasoning becomes even more sophisticated during pregnancy and continues to supercharge a mother's brain at least into her 40s or 50s.[7] If diversity in decision-making groups is a factor in making smart decisions, what can we say about using more of one's brain to understand the world and its challenges?

This is not meant to be an anti-masculine point; quite the contrary, we must get out of the habit of thinking that lifting ourselves up requires us to pull men down. That's zero-sum thinking, which is not in harmony with an embracing, inclusive worldview. The focus here is to understand that, first, bringing in intuition and emotions and what might seem to be random bits of detail during deliberation may be your method of reaching a conclusion. Your ability to access a whole lot more of your brain to make decisions than some other people is a superpower worth honoring and cultivating. Celebrate that!

The catalyst for transformation has always emerged for me because someone was willing to share their experience. Other people's stories provide the spark of creation that allows my brain

---

6   This data is discussed in Zaidi, Zeenat F. "Gender Differences in Human Brain: A Review." *The Open Anatomy Journal* 2.1 (2010).

7   There is some very interesting scholarship being produced on this subject, though not as much as it deserves. One representative example is Duarte-Guterman, Paula, Benedetta Leuner, and Liisa AM Galea. "The Long and Short Term Effects of Motherhood on the Brain." *Frontiers in Neuroendocrinology* 53 (2019): 100740.

to open to possibilities that were previously not in my known reality. We only know what we know at any juncture in our lives. Sometimes, new information and perspectives flow to us, and it is a matter of discerning which ones resonate, and which ones don't. Most of the time, it is about taking ownership, engaging with our curiosity, and daring to question the status quo, which is, in itself, a miracle.

I was raised in the small town of St. Clair, Michigan—population 4,500 when I was living there. There are lovely benefits of growing up in a tight community where everyone knows everyone, but feeling free to think expansively and outside the norm was rarely one of them. As a rural town that was a mix of agriculture, salt mining, and boating, there was little need to explore other places or diverge from the pattern of life passed down from generation to generation. Detroit was only an hour's drive away, but few found the need or desire to venture that far afield.

I usually gravitated toward people who wanted more than this. When I was in grade school, I learned from my babysitter that she was going to transfer to a boarding school because the education at our small-town high school was not challenging her. This sounded exciting! So, when it came time for me to go to high school, I learned that only about 15% of the graduating class went on to a four-year college. I wanted to go to college and did not feel supported in an atmosphere that didn't aspire to do the same.

With the encouragement of my parents and the principal of my elementary school, I explored the idea of going away to school. I chose Mount St. Joseph Academy, an all-girls boarding school in London, Ontario. While the school was only two hours from my home, it exposed me to a variety of cultures and backgrounds (my hometown remains 97% white). I also got the liberating experience of living away from home. My choice to go to boarding school was met with criticism and judgment from my peers and adults. I was called a traitor and asked if I thought

I was too good for everyone there. I created another stir when I went out of state for college.

Despite these hurtful remarks, I knew in my gut I was making a choice that was right for me and my development. Sometimes, following the VOICE framework and rewriting your Mother Codes is uncomfortable for those in our immediate atmosphere. Out of the fear that erupts in them as you venture out into new territory, they may try and pull you down or make degrading comments to keep them from feeling uncomfortable. But I've found that the freedom and healing that come from adopting awareness as a life principle and practice far outweigh the risks and downsides.

Honoring Shifts in Awareness

Cultivating self-awareness as a mother does mean digging into the intricacies of your thoughts, emotions, and reactions as a compass to navigate the complexities of parenting with authenticity. This journey is an invitation to understand your strengths and weaknesses, fostering personal growth that benefits you and has the potential to enrich the connection with your child. It is simple but not easy, and we need as much support along the way as possible.

Throughout my academic and personal development journey, I have found many theorists and practitioners in the fields of psychology, existential philosophy, human development, neuroscience, and more. Some have moved me and provided valuable insights, while others have rocked my world. Collectively, they have had an enormous impact on raising my awareness and broadening my field of vision. There are a number of them that speak deeply regarding awareness in general, but then seen through the lens of motherhood, their ideas and practices reflect a kaleidoscope of opportunities.

I drew inspiration from the work of renowned psychologist Daniel J. Siegell, (particularly his book *Parenting from the Inside Out*). He posits that each nuance of our daily living and the emotions we experience in relationship to our children invite us to look inward for healing of our past hurts. I did not realize how much having a child would stir up old trauma, but to discover this is a good thing and a normal part of the dance of parenthood that sadly remains behind the veil of most people's awareness has been a gift.

With my first daughter, I had a challenging breastfeeding experience. I was not producing an abundance of milk, she was not latching well, my nipples were so very sore, and most distressing, she was not gaining weight. But it was something I had my heart set on, so I wanted to go for it before shifting directions. I did all the usual things—lactation consultant, fenugreek tea, nipple creams—and her weight gain was improving, but far from robust.

I was just about to start adding formula to her feedings when I was coached to first look inside at what nursing and the challenges my daughter and I were having were bringing up for me. I became aware of limiting beliefs I had about myself and my ability to provide and receive nourishment and my fears of growing. When I added this layer of emotional introspection and healing, the door to a broader array of possibilities (which included supplementing with organic half-and-half) became available. The truth is there is no formula for this or any important decision you make regarding nourishing yourself and your loved ones. What I am suggesting is to include your self-awareness and healing. My pediatrician was impressed with my commitment to a deeper exploration and willingness to follow a path, even though it wasn't mainstream yet because it felt right for me and my daughter. I was even invited to talk to a group of his residents. He said they need to hear stories like this so they know what is possible for their patients that goes beyond the routine medical model.

It was a painful and scary process. When your infant isn't gaining weight, the impulse to act, even against your Mother Code, is driven by fear. I had to tune in and give myself some space before deciding to shift course. I had a team around me that I trusted would not let me put myself or our daughter in danger. This let me go deep into my pain surfacing. Dr. Shefali Tsabary, a clinical psychologist and author of *The Conscious Parent*, validates this approach and goes further to say that feeling our pain as parents is useful and *essential*. My release of pain moved me out of lower brain survival thinking and into my frontal lobe, where I could make decisions from my executive functioning. I like to imagine that my unexpressed pain was clogging my milk ducts!

I also felt very seen and understood by Donald Winnicott, a renowned psychoanalyst, when he wrote about his concept of the "good enough mother." His encouragement to be aware not only of my children's needs but also of the importance of my well-being continues to be a message I need to hear repeatedly. This awareness forms the cornerstone of a shame-free nurturing environment where, based on their unique abilities and needs, both mother and child can thrive.

As I continue to share my and other's experience, knowledge, and wisdom to raise your awareness, it is imperative to remember you are always in the driver's seat. You get to immerse in whatever level feels right to you, and ultimately, it is always your choice if, how, and when you put your awareness into action in a way that works for your and your baby's particular needs.

Nurturing Your Intuition

When new information is brought into the foreground and awareness is being raised, you can experience sensations in your body— perhaps your jaw tightens, you have a pang in your gut, your skin itches, or heat rises. This is your body talking to you as a first responder to the data entering your system. Learning to read the language of your body is like unlocking the vault of deeper truths and universal wisdom.

Despite its profound potential, you may feel hesitant or even fearful to reconnect to this innate but lost language of the body. That fear can prevent you from embracing and using your intuitive abilities. This is why I am repeatedly emphasizing its importance, singing its praises, and inviting you to partner with your intuition throughout this book. If I sound like a broken record, it is for good reason. I know intuition is something you understand but living in resonance and congruency with it is work for all of us to engage in.

One of the primary reasons we are afraid to use our intuition is the cultural emphasis on logic, reason, and empirical evidence. From the moment we are born, we are taught to value rational thinking and tangible proof over abstract, intuitive insights. This societal bias toward the masculine energy of rationality leads to distrusting your intuitive senses—especially when the latter is undervalued. When your intuition is often labeled as unreliable or less valid, it makes perfect sense to be reluctant and even tune out the messages and wisdom flowing through your body.

Our current culture of devaluing our intuition is layered with centuries of historical precedents intensifying the instinct to shut out our inner knowing. During the witch hunts of the 15th to 18th centuries, countless women were persecuted, tortured, and executed for exhibiting behaviors deemed unnatural or threatening by a patriarchal society. These women, who often had profound healing abilities, deep understanding of nature, and spiritual insights, were labeled as witches. Their intuition, a source of strength and guidance, was vilified as dark and dangerous. This persecution silenced individual women and instilled a pervasive fear that discouraged others from trusting and expressing their intuitive gifts. This historical trauma has permeated through generations and lives with us today.

Personal insecurities also play a significant role in the reluctance to embrace intuition. Intuition requires us to trust ourselves deeply to have faith in our inner knowing without needing external validation. This level of self-trust can be daunting, especially in a world that constantly bombards us with conflicting information and opinions. The fear of making mistakes or the potential consequences of following an unconventional path can inhibit our willingness to listen to our intuition.

While the horror of how our intuitive power was vilified still runs through our nervous systems, many women stand out against the stifling forces that have kept us silent. We need lots of encouragement and inspiration on the path to claiming our intuitive power. In the words of Oprah Winfrey, "I've trusted the still, small voice of intuition my entire life. And the only time I've made mistakes is when I didn't listen."

As women and mothers, it is our calling to honor and trust our intuition. This divine gift empowers us to nurture, guide, and inspire those around us. By embracing our intuitive wisdom, we not only enrich our own lives and contribute to a more compassionate and balanced world but also play a part in dismantling and breaking the psychic ties to historical trauma. Let us reclaim this sacred connection, unlock the full spectrum of our potential, tap into the Cosmic Codes, and celebrate the profound insights it brings.

I encourage you to include some aspect of claiming the power of your intuition in your rewritten Mother Code. As I said, it's something we grasp cognitively but will need to bathe in it for the trust to rebuild and to reconnect with it. A world where intuition and rationality coexist in harmony is a world I want to live in. And the more I orient to this balanced approach, the more possible it becomes for my daughters and their daughters and sons to come to live in a brighter, more inclusive world.

Awakening Your Power to Choose

Ahhh, "choice"! One of my favorite words of power!

Yes, there are philosophical arguments about whether choice is an illusion or part of our free will, but that is more of a distraction than a useful distinction. One of our uniquely human behaviors is the ability to make choices. From where those choices arise and how conscious we are when we make them is an interesting inquiry. Our instincts do not run our every action, and while we are highly programmed by our families and culture, we still can step outside our wiring to make our own individual choices. Rewriting the Mother Code is about making discerned choices, choices made after we have allowed space for our curiosity to be satiated. After we have done our due diligence around the landscape of mothering, we become aware that there exists a playground full of choices. From there, you can feel and intuit your way into choices that resonate with your Mother Code.

Simone de Beauvoir's existential wisdom, echoed in *The Second Sex* (1949), casts the act of choice in the mystical light of self-discovery. The goddess within guides women through a labyrinth of choices, acknowledging the sacred responsibility of shaping one's maternal destiny. Choices become sacred rites, keys to unlocking the mysteries of the divine dance of motherhood.

I find it maddening that we dedicate so much time, expense, and effort to studying and planning for our careers. We put focus and attention on getting into a good college, and in more privileged households a lot of money is spent on test prep and consultants to increase the possibility of getting into a top school. There are myriad personality and other tests that show what careers we are best-suited for. Yet, with something as profound and life-altering as parenting, we treat it as a binary choice.

As I mentioned earlier, the "Yes" I want to be a parent or "No" I do not want to be a parent declaration is alive and well in our culture. That we can even say no is a recent and still provocative choice. The point is we are not accustomed to thinking much about the choices that surround our mothering choices.

I coached a couple who decided not to become parents of children. It was a challenging and painful decision, but as they embraced it, they found deep meaning and pleasure in many ways, including their careers and relationship. In seeing them experience profound joy in the life they were creating and living, I felt a pang of jealousy. I realized that my choice meant a significant sacrifice of energy and resources that would be spent caring for and raising my children. That energy could have gone into my marriage, career, and other pursuits. It felt heretical to even have this thought. How dare I ponder regretting having children! Does that mean I don't love them or wish I didn't have them? No, I feel secure in my love for my daughters, and I chose this path with as much clarity as I could at the time. This is about acknowledging the full truth of our experience and taking responsibility for our choices—all aspects of it.

We are not victims, and no matter what situation we find ourselves in on our mothering journey, especially the ones where choices are restricted due to bureaucratic policies, we always have the power to choose our internal state. Our choices stretch beyond our personal experience. I was not aware of it, but my quest for unconventional conception and birth experiences was not just a choice that resonated with me but a feminist stance against medical practices that often focus on convenience and money over a woman's agency and empowered experience.

REFLECTION

Think about something or someone that is causing you stress or worry. Now picture yourself in your home or office or wherever or with whoever is the source of your upset. Next, imagine yourself floating up to the ceiling and observing this upset from this distance. Notice what you feel when you do this.

From there, float yourself up above the space you are in—above your house or office. Observe from this vantage point: What happens to your experience of the upset? What emotions do you notice?

Keep doing this—taking yourself above your neighborhood, then above your state, then your country, then way up in the sky on the edge of the Earth's atmosphere.

Last, take yourself up into the cosmos where you can see not just Earth, but the sun and all the planets and moons in our solar system.

Notice your experience at each level.

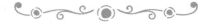

Let me tell you the story of a family of three generations of women studying the Mother Code without naming it as such. The first was Emily Fogg Mead, who, upon learning in 1901 that she was pregnant, began a diary scrupulously detailing her daily activity based on her theory that these factors would influence her child's development. Even after that child, a girl, was born, she continued taking notes, eventually filling an additional thirteen notebooks about the activities of her baby girl. That child was Margaret Mead, maybe the most progressive, controversial, and forward-thinking anthropologist of her generation, if not of all time.

Much of Margaret's research and scholarship could be described, without a stretch, as an analysis of the Mother Code, and in her letters to her family and closest friends, she speaks with skepticism of the claims of science at the time about a future "in which all the nurseries have rounded corners and science was going to solve every problem."[8] Margaret's own daughter, Mary Catherine Bateson, also became an anthropologist and eventually wrote a memoir and something like an anthropological study of

---

8   You can read Margaret Mead's letter to her sister at https://www.themarginalian. org/2015/11/30/margaret-mead-elizabeth-letter/.

her parents. What is clear from even a casual browse of the work of these women is that they each built on the work of their mother in rewriting their Mother Codes.

It is no coincidence that one of Margaret Mead's most famous quotes is, "Never doubt that a small group of thoughtful, committed citizens can change the world; indeed, it's the only thing that ever has." In her own life, she experienced the power of the work of such groups and made herself an active part of them, including across generations. To you I say, never doubt in the power of a small group of women who have rewritten their Mother Codes to change the world; it is only such groups of people who ever have.

As we stand amid feminist narratives, academic analyses, goddess whispers, and the mystical embrace of the divine feminine, we see the unveiling of the cosmic tapestry of motherhood. The threads intertwine, creating a rich tableau where dismantling internalized dialogues, empowerment through knowledge, and mystical experiences converge. As we continue this journey, you will dig deeper into these possibilities, exploring how your VOICE can amplify your inner wisdom and empower you to continuously rewrite your Mother Code to navigate the challenges of motherhood with consciousness and rebellion.

Raising your awareness of the power that resides in you and how power has been silenced, awakening and honoring your intuition alongside the doubts and fears that can arise, and choosing *your* path because even under your discerning scrutiny it feels so aligned with your new vision for yourself—this is embracing the cosmic side of mothering. This is soaring to the highest heights while also staying grounded in the truth of your embodied experience. This is opening yourself to the magic that happens when you let go of the belief that safety sits inside of control. The sooner you realize control is an illusion, the sooner you can experience the loving compassion and empowerment of the universe.

Prior to writing the conclusion of this chapter, I pulled the perfect oracle card from the *Vision Quest Tarot*, by Gayan Sylvie Winter and Jo Dose.[9] It was the "Four of Earth—Security" that said: "Accepting our absolute insecurity is the only way to remain safe. So, learn to rest in apparent insecurity. Begin to recognize the unchanging power in every change, every new and different situation. In this welcoming acceptance, you find the security that knows no change."

If you are anything like me, you may need to read it several times and let it sink in. It feels so foreign, yet so right. I call it fem-speak, and while it is profoundly contrary to our material and linear-based thinking, it also strikes a chord of truth I want to return home to.

This is your unique journey. This path takes you into the depths of your interior landscape and skyrockets you into the vastness of the dark universe. No one else's journey will mimic yours. At the same time, even in our isolating culture that glorifies individuality, you are not meant to travel this road alone. Our experience as mothers in all of its manifestations is a bond we share, and the golden threads connecting us include both our joy and our pain. Let's celebrate each new awareness and let them ignite the fire of a new paradigm of mothering—one that burns brighter and brighter as each woman adds her flame.

---

9 The entire deck is filled with nuggets of insight like this. Winter, Gayan Silvie, and Jo Dose. *Vision Quest Tarot*. AGM-Urania, Cards edition, 1999.

Rite of Passage—Second Trimester

Our second trimester of growing together, in some ways, may be the most difficult. There has been a lot of information in the chapters, and I have challenged you to dig deep into the Mother Code that has been imprinted on you by family and the broader society. You have written your own Mother Code.

Wow! That is some big, juicy work!

Just like in the second trimester of pregnancy, you are "showing." There is no hiding the fact you are pregnant because your body is miraculously expanding to encompass this new being. There is also no hiding that you have expanded your conscious awareness! Sooo much growth is happening with your baby. Lungs develop, kicking is felt, hearing develops and responds to your voice and fingerprints, and brain development continues—specifically the senses. By the end of the second trimester eyes, that were fused shut are opening. A baby can live outside the womb by the end of this trimester.

How wonderous is it that the development of your baby is beautifully synchronized with *your* development as a mother! Your lungs have developed, and they are breathing air into your VOICE. Your eyes have been opened to the restricting reality of the prevailing Mother Codes. By kicking out old norms and claiming your values and principles, you are making your true self known. Your rewritten Mother Code, like your fingerprint, is uniquely yours. No one else has or will ever have the same one. You are tuning into your senses and connecting with the power of your intuition.

While giving yourself more time in the protective and nourishing space of the womb, you are also capable of emerging into the world and living your Mother Code.

This is all a big deal! In your first trimester, you entered territory that was new to you in some ways. In this second trimester, you pushed to start making the changes in your perception and thought processes that lead to transformation. With growth comes discomfort. You have likely found some uncomfortable passages and your awareness was raised as to the impact of some unpleasant memories, maybe even things you haven't thought about for years. And now you've made an affirmative declaration about who you are and where you are going.

More and more, you are affirming and nurturing your intuitive senses. You are poised to make choices that are harmonious with your head and your heart.

I won't say it gets easier from here, but if you've been stretching muscles you rarely use (and that will be true for more readers than not), just know the more you use them, the easier it gets and the richer the results will be. So now we begin stepping into what this new way of being looks like and feels like for you, as well as how to accelerate its development and how to avoid pitfalls. You are developing a practice, just as athletes or musicians or artists develop their method. Let's talk about your routine. Let's talk about tools. Let's talk about your state of mind. And perhaps as important as developing your system, we will talk about connecting to the worldwide community of people engaged in the same journey, as well as fellow travelers.

You are moving into a whole new world. Let's begin!

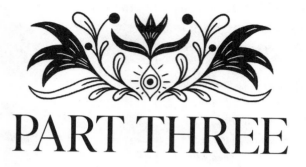

PART THREE

THIRD TRIMESTER

The dark forest isn't a scary place.
It is fecund, pulsing with life,
Womb
that we have been taught to fear.
The physical pain of childbirth is a lie
we have been lulled into believing.
Wait, what? How can something so real
in our bodies
be a lie?
Did Nothingness feel pain when Universe was created?
Women were not punished with the pain of childbirth.
The glory of the ecstatic experience was taken from us.
Or more likely
we gave it freely
for the greater good or need at the time.
We no longer need to live that false reality.

Only women have the power to reclaim it.
Conception, pregnancy, birth are a cosmic phenomenon.
The trinity of wholeness,
of holiness.

Why would an experience of union of
 divine feminine and
divine masculine
that sends ripples of ecstatic pleasure throughout our bodies,
that breaks us open with beautiful and
wild and
unleashed sensations;
an unhinging where we utter the sounds of the universe,
"Ahhh...ohhh...Oh My God!"
not unfold in that same manner?

Chapter 7
A New Set of Codes

We mother how we live.

If we orient our lives toward seeing life only through the lens of crisis, control, convenience, comfort, and coping, we close ourselves off from what lies on the other side and beyond. Releasing control and being shattered by an experience can have a transformative effect. There were times in my birth labors when I thought I might split open, but then, at a certain point, all that ego-based self gave way to a transcendent moment where I became birth itself.

Is this the spiritual birth of woman into mother?

All the wonders of the world are born through cycles of destruction and renewal and rebirth—some through a sudden event like a meteor hitting the Earth, most others through the process of being part of an evolving universe. Our Earth is a living entity that has been around for some 4.5 billion years and is continuously birthing. We are learning the hard way that there is no controlling her ongoing emergence. Our inability to not play well with her and mirror and merge with her ways could lead to our death. Following this cataclysm, a new evolution of species will emerge, and Mother Earth will carry on her merry way. I don't want my daughters' or my daughters' future children to suffer through an avoidable death of a human epoch.

I have hope we can alter our species' trajectory and instead show how capable we are of reattuning and acknowledging our connection to Mother Earth and the infinite universe in which she resides.

On my recent travel to Iceland, I was struck by how eminently apparent it is that the Earth comes before and after us. With reverence and awe, I affectionately call the landscape of Iceland in-your-face raw beauty! It is also a land of extremes. I experienced daylight that merely ebbed into dusk but never really ended, waterfalls at every turn (there are over 10,000 in Iceland), freezing cold ocean water lapping onto beaches littered with mini-icebergs, and soothingly warm water flowing up from springs and rivers over 6,000 feet below the earth's surface.

While the whole island is vibrating with energy, the location that called out to me was the Snæfellsjökull glacier (don't ask me to pronounce it!). This is touted to have a major earth energy vortex—like the ones said to lie within the earth in Egypt or Sedona, AZ. My heart tugged, and I knew this was where I must go on my solo excursion!

The closer my guide got me to the glacier, the more I felt like a child coming home to her mother—only not my biological mother but The Mother. I don't have words for this experience. Despite the glacier being massive in size, I felt like I could hug her. I nestled into an indent in the rough landscape that somehow felt like a warm embrace. Some cultures, such as the original peoples in the Americas, don't just call certain mountains *symbols* of a divine mother– they *are* the Divine Mother. A living entity. And while I have cognitively understood this, I now have an inkling of the embodied experience of it.

Volcanic activity is present throughout the country in many ways and stages! Holy eruptions! How much more feminine can we get? The fiery red magma ebbs, flows, and pours out from deep within the womb of this Earth Mother. Her flow is anything but subtle! It is movement! It pulses with a force that destroys anything in the way of her creative intention to birth new earth. Some eruptions release harmful gasses and blankets of ash—both of which have the combined effect of destruction and damage, as well as providing the components for future sustainability and growth. I realized that rewriting our Mother Codes—childhood and cultural—are the tectonic plates that shift to create the conditions for the eruption and giving way to new possibilities that were hidden below the surface until the circumstances were just right to bring them forth.

It is not a coincidence that I journeyed to Iceland while I engaged in writing and editing this book. My sense that we are microcosms of the Earth was validated as I, too, felt cracked open and a creative force like none I had experienced flowed through me and poured onto the pages. This experience affirms my belief that as we have distanced ourselves from the natural rhythms of nature, we have limited our access to living the human life we came from the cosmos to Earth to live.

The reward of doing the hard work of plumbing the depths of our inner landscape and cracking open to create new realities is the possibility of soaring into the realms of the infinite cosmos. Sitting with the potential of connecting with the vastness of the universe is both thrilling and, to be honest, terrifying. But the more I have turned toward this reality, the more guided, supported, and connected to myself and others I feel. I have had so many moments over the last couple of years where I chuckle at the coincidences and blessings that continue to come my way. I am sure there are so many I have missed as I learn to embrace this new outlook, but as these graces become more woven into the fabric of my daily living, I never take them for granted, and my gratitude for them increases.

My experience leads me to believe this outpouring of blessings from the Universe combines opening myself to Source and choosing to have faith in moments of doubt and uncertainty. Choosing full faith is like surrendering to the current of the river, such that even when you smash into the rocks, you understand that it is the nature of existence. I cannot blame the rocks for being there, but I can learn, and I can appreciate what they reveal. That I am a spiritual being having a human experience has become a growing part of my rewritten Mother Code.

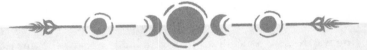

SURRENDER RITUAL

It is possible to cultivate a relationship with the Sacred Feminine. Whether this is something you are considering for the first time or you are at a place of deepening your current relationship with Her, I offer this meditation to move it forward.

Place your hands over your heart, feeling its steady rhythm, the source of your life force. Close your eyes and envision a soft, radiant light glowing within your chest. This light represents the Divine Feminine, a nurturing and powerful presence that resides within you. As you connect with this light, speak aloud, or in your mind, these words:

"I surrender myself fully and completely to the security of Your embrace."

Feel the weight of the world lift from your shoulders as you speak these words. Imagine yourself being held in the loving and protective arms of the Divine Mother, secure and safe. Next, place one hand on your heart and

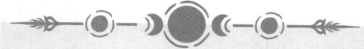

the other on your lower abdomen, connecting your heart and your womb, the centers of love and creation. Continue with the next affirmation:

"I share all of me with You as Your dedicated daughter, sister, friend."

As you say this, feel a deep connection to the Divine Feminine, knowing you are her cherished child, a sister in spirit, and a friend who walks in her light. Feel her presence surrounding you, supporting you, and accepting all that you are. Finally, open your arms wide, as if embracing the world, and speak the final affirmation:

"I live my day with passion and integrity in service of the Divine Feminine so that all may know You."

As you declare this, feel the energy of purpose and passion infusing your entire being. Visualize yourself moving through your day with self-efficacy, grace, and dedication, spreading the love and wisdom of the Divine Feminine in all that you do.

After speaking these phrases, take a moment to stand in stillness, letting the energy settle into your body and mind. When you feel ready, bring your hands back to your heart, take a deep breath, and slowly open your eyes. Carry the essence of these affirmations with you throughout your day, knowing you are always held in the embrace of the Divine Feminine and that your actions reflect Her love and power.

(Note: Adapt these words in a way that aligns with your belief system to surrender to and partner with a loving G-d, source, energy, or earthly support.)

Cosmic Codes

In full transparency, I went through a discernment process on whether I should use "cosmic" so overtly in this book. I know I risk alienating some potential readers, and despite earning a doctorate and being research-based, I will be written off as unserious. My inquiry around this judgment has led me to the realization that the rejection of the quest for intuitive growth and spirituality is another attempt to minimize and degrade the Yin concept of being unfathomably vast and seeking connection with the Divine in ourselves and others.

By embracing cosmic, I intend to deflate any limiting conjectures that come between me and my embodied potential! So, let's go all in—into the infinite possibilities of the cosmic. I encourage your full immersion, but as always, the choice of your level of surrender into this space is all yours.

At the risk of over-simplifying and putting into language that which defies the constraints of the written word, I offer a space to contemplate and envision expansive possibilities. Consider these five Cosmic Codes as a starting point on your journey into your inner sanctuary. Loosen your grip on your conscious and comfortable reality, fall into the abyss of your emptiness, and discover the wonders of your being.

First Cosmic Code: You are a Mother

You are a mother!
You conceive.
You create.
You birth.

For people who have physical wombs, you have within you a sacred container that holds the potential to provide sanctuary for a soul's transition into the earthly realm. All women have the womb capacity to grow dreams, incubate ideas, nurture relationships, cultivate careers, and so much more.

Anywhere you focus your care, concern, emotional labor, and love, you are mothering. It could be a moment of appreciating the beauty of a tiny flower, leading a work team in a project, supporting an aging parent, or getting on the floor and playing with your child—in these acts, you are accessing the mother energy of gratitude, awe, caring, loving, and guiding.

By identifying with mother energy, you reduce the risk of losing yourself in a narrowly defined role. Instead, you gain a superpower that you can apply to all areas of your life and throughout your whole time living and breathing on this earth. Imagine moving from a cubbyhole experience of life in a preprogrammed identity to one that takes flight and soars far and high.

Through this cosmic code, you also break free of illusionary silos that separate you by roles or any choice you make on your mothering journey. Our intersection in the awareness, acceptance, and actualization of mother energy breaks a divide that has fractured our collective power as women. You are a creator. Recognize yourself as an original creator, and when you do, any lingering doubts of your power and potential will fade into the shadows. The breadth and depth of your creative power reveals itself in the ordinary and the extraordinary. You create beauty. You create connection. You create life.

You are a destroyer. Women are inherently attuned to the creative and destructive cycles of life. Own this power and wield it thoughtfully. Like the universe and volcanoes, birth and death are not linear events; they are part of the flow and constant movement of all that is. You know this as truth.

Second Cosmic Code: Pain Is Your Portal

Your Pain is interwoven with pleasure.
Your Pain is a conduit to altered states.
Your Pain is sacred and divine.

I used to ascribe to the well-trod theory that humans are designed to move away from pain toward pleasure in a straight line. Au contraire—pain and pleasure are not on a linear continuum; they are inextricably interwoven together! In a culture that fears pain and fails to honor pain's wisdom, we would be compelled to move as far away from it as possible. This theory, in which our range of sight is narrowed by a patriarchal monocle, cannot grasp the more expansive truth that pain is nothing more than cosmic energy in one of its many manifestations.

Sexual intercourse, for example, sits on the razor's edge of pain and pleasure. It is messy, primal, and raw. It is ecstatic. To orgasm is to release accumulated energy and lose control of our temporal reality. It can be terrifying to fully surrender into the abyss and ride the wave from beginning to end. It requires a space of safety and trust to go there. You are the owner of this experience. You are responsible for your pleasure—both in asking for what you want and in creating an atmosphere of mutual consent. Under those conditions, you become aware of the wings that carry you as far as you are willing to go. When we see pain as an integral part of the cycle of creative and destructive processes, our fear of it decreases, we move into acceptance, and eventually we learn to welcome pain in our experience.

I was terrified of scuba diving. My paralyzing fear of death by drowning has kept this activity off my bucket list! My husband's suggestion that our family all get certified in diving coincided with the diaphragmic breathwork and bodywork sessions I was engaged in. During the sessions I was tuning into my capacity to breathe even when it was restricted or difficult. I realized that despite limited airflow, I could still breathe.

"What was I thinking saying yes to this?" I thought as I contemplated doing the unfathomable and going on my first dive. I could barely sleep the night before and I almost backed out but went for it and took it one step at a time. In the first two dives, most of my attention was focused on the many discomforts and fear of all the things that could go wrong I barely looked around me. "Why was it so easy and carefree for my husband and daughters?" I wondered. When I asked my husband how he was managing it so effortlessly, he said, "It's not easy at all. I have the same issues and discomfort you are describing; I just accept them as part of the experience." Whoa, this blew me away! I decided to adopt his philosophy on my last dive, and for the first time, I was overcome by the incredible beauty and other worldliness of life under the water.

It was such a huge lesson for me to step into my fear of potential pain and accept the interconnected nature of pain and pleasure. If I had forgone the experience, it would have been a valid choice, but in moving into it, a completely new world was revealed to me.

Oh, what glorious experiences are born from pain!

Third Cosmic Code: You Are a Vessel of Love

You are love.

Love is ever present in you.

Love flows from you.

What a wondrous experience love is! Throughout time humans have tried to capture the essence of it in poetry, song, and prose. It is impossible! But we catch glimpses and we continue to wrap our minds and hearts around it in earnest. The simple truth is this— LOVE IS. It is difficult for us to settle into something that is 100% accepting and being. Love is also 100% who you are.

Remember, there is a reason that a dominant influence would not want us to know that at our core, we are—love. If you become programmed to believe that love needs to be earned or given to you, then the power and blessings love holds will always be out of reach and in someone else's hands.

I will not preach or pretend to have mastered love, but I will say that by choosing to be on the journey of claiming that I am a vessel of love I experience more abundance than lack. It helps me stay out of victimhood—or at least notice when I am in it faster—and this is a wondrous experience.

To aim for understanding instead of blame is a loving act. To be curious is to be free. To come from a place of personal responsibility when I hold others accountable to live true to their values is acting from love.

Imagine a world where more and more of us do the personal work to move beyond the platitudes and ego-centered behavior mistakenly claiming to come from love. Instead, we encounter life in all the raw, honest, complex, unpredictable, and wonderful realities with emotional responsibility. That is a world whose beating heart pulses with the lifeblood of love. That is a world where love is our foundation individually and collectively. Every loving act contributes to the creation of this world.

Choose to be the love that you are.

Fourth Cosmic Code: You Are Part of a Greater Whole

You are one with a loving universe!
You are never alone.
You matter.

The universe is not outside of you. The universe resides inside of you. The universe *is* you. When you doubt we are all connected, or that you are made of stardust or that you are part of an expanding universe, I am here to remind you it is encoded in our physiology. Dr. Jill Bolte Taylor's work on Whole Brain Living has confirmed that our capacity to experience ourselves as energy and connect with an all-loving universe is facilitated through an area of your brain.[1] Thus, the belief that the universe is out there somewhere or that you are alone is an illusion. Being one with the infinite universe doesn't just feel like the truth that it is, it is scientific fact. Let that sink in. Let that blow the circuits of your former programming.

---

1 Dr. Bolte Taylor's work is nothing less than groundbreaking. You can learn more about her at https://www.drjilltaylor.com/. It was my great pleasure to talk with her and share the conversation on my podcast; you can hear our discussion at https://podcasts.apple. com/us/podcast/whole-brain-living-with-dr-jill-bolte-taylor/id1534581166?i=1000565404520.

We are intrinsically connected to the universe profoundly and fascinatingly: We are made from its matter. This concept, often summed up by the phrase "we are stardust," reflects the enduring connection between human beings and the cosmos. The story begins in the hearts of stars, where nuclear fusion creates the elements necessary for life.

In the cores of ancient stars, hydrogen atoms fused to form helium, and through subsequent fusion processes, heavier elements like carbon, oxygen, and iron were born. When these stars reached the end of their lifespans, they often exploded in spectacular supernovae, scattering these elements across the universe. This cosmic debris eventually coalesced into new stars, planets, and everything on them—including us.

Our planet, Earth, formed from the remnants of these stellar explosions. The elements that make up our bodies—carbon in our cells, calcium in our bones, iron in our blood—were all forged in the furnaces of ancient stars. This means that the matter we are composed of has an origin story that spans billions of years and vast distances in space. Our existence is tied to the grand, ongoing story of the universe. It's a beautiful reminder of our shared origins and the intricate web of matter and energy that links us to the cosmos.

Are you ready for another mind-expanding concept? Here it is...You are never alone. You always have community within you. It is crowded in there! With the echoes of your direct human lineage combined with the matter and energy of all time and space that are your heritage, it is not a matter of if you are alone, it is more what aspects of your lineage do you want to befriend and commune with!

Do you value any of the following: the welfare of the greater good? Cooperation? Compassion? If you answered yes to any of these, then whether you are aware of it or not, research shows you share the attributes of people who believe in the oneness of the universe. Imagine a world where everyone embraces these qualities.

And what if we understood that when we show hate or judgment toward anyone or anything, we are inflicting that negativity directly onto ourselves because we are all connected?

The ripple effects that correlate with this truth are daunting, I understand. There is tremendous responsibility knowing your thoughts and deeds don't just impact you. They impact everyone and everything on the planet and beyond. Whoa—no wonder we are inclined to ignore this reality! Trust me, this is not just another way for us to feel guilty when we are not living our highest values. When you shift perspective and look through the lens of how much you matter, a much more loving and positive image takes shape.

Fifth Cosmic Code: Mothering Yourself Is a Sacred Experience

You are safe and held in the arms of a loving Mother.
You are wise beyond measure.
You have everything you need inside of you for nourishment and healing.

What is it to mother oneself? It is as simple as bathing in a compliment and as deep as doing the internal work to heal past trauma. Everything and everyone that you encounter has the potential to provide self-mothering—if we choose it to be. There is nourishment found in both the bleakest of circumstances and the most abundant and beautiful. It is yours to find them within everything, some of which will sometimes feel contradictory.

Self-mothering is not a time-based experience. Awareness and tuning into the present moment do not exist in our linear time construct. This is consciousness and engagement with all that is. Engaging in activities that foster deeper connection and pleasure with yourself for moments or months is and always will be time well spent.

Our internal loving mother resides in every cell, every thought, every heartbeat. There is a never-ending supply of affirmation, encouragement, hopefulness, and positive intentions, to name a few.

There is no reason to ever feel scarce regarding self-mothering. A reservoir of inner nourishment is infinitely available to you. And to be clear, every human on the planet deserves resource abundance. This is a critical issue for the collective to solve.

While there is ongoing abundance, you will tend to and care for your inner garden, and when you do so, it will provide nourishment and growth not only for yourself but for those around you. Grow your tree of self-love and the flowers, fruits, and seeds it fosters are available to those around you. Be the mycelium and the rivers and the mountains and the dirt and the acorns. Be the sky and the stars and the aurora borealis. Feast on the banquet that is you!

Trust the wisdom that resides within you. Our being is a vessel of truth, beauty, love, and wisdom. Focus your attention on the powerful physical, emotional, cognitive, and spiritual mechanisms that align with this truth. When you tune into the highest frequencies of each aspect of you, what you need in any moment will be immediately clear. The alchemic synergy of these forces will guide your thoughts, decisions, and actions.

Rediscovering Our Emotional Essence

When accessing and living the Cosmic Codes, your emotions are your superpowers. Like any super heroine on her quest, you need to first know you have this power, then learn to express it—testing its boundaries—and then acquire the skills to focus and channel its power for your and humanity's highest good. Sound fun? Or at least intriguing? I hope so!!

Fortunately, you don't need a genetically modified spider to bite you or to land here from another planet to have your own powers, you are born with them! This is never clearer than when you spend time with a baby. Have you ever noticed that when a baby comes into the room how all the attention goes toward them? How is it that this being that doesn't speak, cannot do anything productive other than eat, sleep, pee, and poop, captivates us so intensely? Yes, they smell amazing, and their disproportionately large head size compared to body size makes them extra cute, but it is more than that—it is their full presence and raw expression of their emotions that hold such incredible power.

So, what happens? Why would we lower the volume on, mute, and even turn off our emotions and act as if we don't even possess them if they are so powerful? The answer is complex, but at the root is our current family and cultural programming. Emotions are full of Yin energy, and they are too messy for our civilized world; so if the intention is for Yang power to dominate our culture, then muting emotional expression makes sense. The attempts to tame them so we could keep order in the chaos of evolutionary development has swung too far in one direction.

Our family atmosphere is also a powerful source of dampening emotional expression. I know this well, as it was not safe to express my feelings in my home, and I learned to not exist emotionally. When I started group and individual therapy, I waited for permission to eke out a tear. People would point out that my throat and upper chest would turn bright red because I was repressing my tears. I would smile when I was angry. My body was compensating and paying the price for my refusal to open myself and flow with my emotions.

I had to unlearn all I had been taught about emotions so I could regain access to and expression of my full range of emotions. This was challenging work, but over time, the reclamation of my emotional essence took shape. Rather than avoid them at all costs, they have become both a portal into divine connection with myself and others and a pragmatic necessity to keeping a clean and clear internal house. I have learned that while I may never be comfortable with anger, having access to it when I need it reflects the power of requisite variety in our emotional tool kit. I cannot emphasize this enough, so I will say it again. Requisite variety with our emotions gives us power. Silence and emotional repression cause us physical harm and cut us off from a core part of our being.

I had a big wakeup call that drove this point home during an incident with my daughter, Morgan, on Michigan Avenue in Chicago. Morgan was seven at the time, and Hannah, her sister, was five. Following a day of shopping on the Magnificent Mile we were all walking back to our car a couple blocks away. When we crossed the busy street, I assumed my mother or my husband had their eye on Morgan while I was holding Hannah's hand. Once across the street and walking down the block I realized Morgan wasn't with us. Panic and terror ran through my body. A parent's worst nightmare! We all looked around. I ran to the traffic officer in the road and said my daughter was lost. After what seemed like an eternity but was only a couple minutes, we spotted her on a nearby corner with a young couple. I felt so fortunate that it was a kind couple who she approached to say she was separated from us. We thanked them profusely, hugged Morgan like crazy, and affirmed her in how she handled the situation.

Once I calmed down and we were home safe, I was filled with the devastating realization that during that whole time, I never once yelled for her or cried out her name as we searched for her. My mechanism to freeze my emotions during real or perceived danger, as well as the historical belief it was not okay to be messy or make a fuss, overrode the response to do whatever it took to find my daughter. I have yet to forgive myself for this, but I have found compassion, and I redoubled my efforts to build the muscles of emotional requisite variety.

I am heartened to see that it is becoming more mainstream to value and foster emotional intelligence. We have a long way to go, however, to rewrite the codes that bind us to both the general and gender-related biases our culture holds around what is considered acceptable expression of emotions. The more we individually take responsibility for our corner of the world, the more it will become the new normal.

Whether you are beginning your journey of rediscovering your emotional essence or at some phase of deepening your connection with them, it is a muscle that offers so many gifts as we continue to strengthen it.

REFLECTION:

Consider that any time you connect emotionally with yourself and others, you are uniting the uniquely human experience with the cosmic. The more we open ourselves to our emotional experience, the more we open ourselves to experience unity with the Divine.

In the spirit of developing these muscles, in your day today, pause and recall one time when you felt each emotion. You can do this in your thoughts, you can journal about it, and you can do it in community with one or more people.

Where did I feel fear today?

Where did I feel hurt today?

Where did I feel anger today?

Where did I feel sadness today?

Where did I feel joy today?

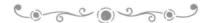

We are all on a journey home to ourselves. Our emotions fuel this journey and reconnect us with the cosmic essence of who we are. As you reclaim the lost pieces of a self that emerged from your mother's womb whole and complete, remember the holiness of your being. The sacred honor of being a vessel for another spirit's journey demands that your first responsibility be to yourself and only then to what you choose to mother.

And so, it is.

So it is that you are a mother.

So it is that your pain is a portal.

So it is that that you are a vessel of love.

So it is that you are connected to a greater whole.

So it is that mothering yourself is a sacred experience.

And so it is that you are all of this and more. Your mothering journey truly has infinite possibilities and can take infinite forms. Knowing this will take you into places you would not have even thought to consider before and let you recognize the many treasures that may have gone unnoticed.

Chapter 8

Living YOUR Mother Code

Let's return to the image of you as a prism, letting the light of the world pass through you and transforming it into radiant colors. Picture yourself in the center of a ring of light and color, with bands of various vivid hues flowing out from inside of you. Now imagine that as you concentrate on any particular color, it glows and increases in volume. You can switch from one color to another in a split second. It is effortless and beautiful, and it is all flowing from you.

Every band of light is another aspect of the Mother Code. What comes to us as a single beam of white light is not a unity but an illusion of something intact, created through dense and complex messaging that begins before you are born. Your innate powers divide the simple light into a complex rainbow and return all the elements of the Code to their original, malleable form, and from this, you create your own Mother Code in the moment. If you wish to focus on your emotions and their value, validity, and the importance of expressing them, imagine this is in the violet spectrum. As you focus on it, it grows and becomes brighter. You can celebrate yourself and the healing power you bring into the world by freely feeling and sharing your emotions. Now, shift to a vision of your child's birth. This may be a deep red band of light. Bask in your vision of that birth and its cosmic significance.

Every aspect of your Mother Code can be incorporated into this exercise. Remember always that each facet of the life you envision for yourself is as accessible as that prism inside of you and that you can visit all facets of your vision in this way. The present and future you are building for yourself are at hand today, and you can access them with a simple thought.

In this third trimester of the book, attempting the exercises or starting the suggested practices, such as journaling or creating art that expresses your journey, places you in the category of living your Mother Code. The rewriting is well underway, and the embodiment has begun. Even as you are reading this page, your neurons are firing differently; new pathways are being built in which your new habits of thought will travel, while the old pathways are increasingly less defined and will grow weaker and weaker. With your engagement and your dedication, you are changing yourself physically. Isn't that amazing?

Another remarkable thing is also taking place: How you are changing is being absorbed by your children and others around you. The mind of a child is an incredible phenomenon, and they pick up everything with a sophistication that goes well beyond simple, conscious, discursive thought. They are growing into the children of a rewritten Mother Code mom, somebody who has taken her identity and her destiny into her hands. And this will only benefit them.

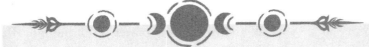

ELEMENTAL RITUAL

Creating practices that bring us in contact with the rhythms of nature and the elements nourish us and protect us from the stress and strain of living in our human bodies. Taking even a few minutes a day goes a long way in building a spiritual practice.

Find a quiet space where you can be alone and centered. If possible, have a candle nearby to represent the element of Fire, and ensure you're in a place where you can comfortably breathe and reflect. Ground yourself, feeling the connection between your body and the Earth beneath you.

Begin by taking a deep, mindful breath of Air, inhaling through your nose and exhaling through your mouth, allowing yourself to arrive in this sacred space.

Gratitude and Connection to Earth:

Place your hands gently on the ground or imagine your hands resting on the Earth, connecting you to its solid, nurturing presence. Speak aloud:

"I am grateful for all that Mother Earth provides, and I acknowledge my need of Her."

Feel the strength and stability of the Earth beneath you, supporting you in every moment. Let this connection ground you, providing a solid foundation from which to grow and flourish.

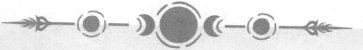

Inspiration and Air:

Bring your attention to your breath, feeling the air as it flows in and out of your lungs. Visualize the air filling your body with energy and light. As you breathe deeply, say:

"I breathe in Air for inspiration and energy."

Imagine the air invigorating your mind and spirit, filling you with clarity, creativity, and the vitality to pursue your path. Feel this energy coursing through you, awakening every part of your being.

Transformation and Fire:

If you have a candle or incense, light it now, or simply visualize a flame burning brightly before you. Gaze at the flame and let its warmth inspire a sense of transformation within you. Speak these words:

"I see this Flame as a symbol of my transformation today."

As you watch the flame flicker and dance, imagine it burning away old patterns, fears, and doubts, making way for new growth, strength, and wisdom. Know that, like the flame, you are ever-changing, transforming into your highest self.

Flow and Water:

Finally, place your hands over your heart, feeling the steady rhythm of your life force. Imagine the gentle flow of water, representing your emotions and experiences. Speak

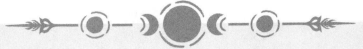

either or both of these affirmations as they resonate with you:

"I am a vessel of Your creation; may I flow with life."

Feel yourself becoming one with the natural flow of life, trusting in the wisdom of your emotions and your experiences. Allow yourself to move gracefully with the currents of life, knowing the Divine Feminine supports you in every moment.

Sit for a moment in silence, feeling the connection with the elements and the Divine Feminine. When you are ready, take a final deep breath, extinguish the flame (if you have lit one), and carry this sense of connection and gratitude with you throughout your day.

Living in Alignment with Your Mother Code

Your Mother Code is your ally, your teacher, your best friend, and your sacred portal to cosmic consciousness. It is divine poetry that guides you through your mountain of pain. It is the spirit of the wind that carries you as you sail on your ocean of emotions. It is the spark that ignites your desires as you become a woman on fire. This isn't something you experience only at church or while you meditate on top of a mountain. On the contrary, your Mother Code statement opens the door to enlightened experiences from the profound to the mundane.

It is with you as you are deciding if you even want to have children or not. It is there for you during a heated discussion with your company about paid time off and when you are once again picking up toys scattered all over the living room.

It takes active engagement to realize your Mother Code's potential. You are building an intimate relationship with your Cosmic Codes, and it will have all the same aspects of a human couple—from the initial excitement and honeymoon phase to the nitty-gritty of navigating commitment, to nourishing it to grow over the long term. Whether your statement explicitly states it, I know that by creating it, you have made a promise to mother yourself first. You are providing the best possible environment for anyone you choose to include in your life—friends, spouse/partner, children, pets.

If you feel a little squirmy at the idea of creating an intimate relationship with some words on a piece of paper, I will remind you that your Mother Code is nothing more than a reflection of *you* put into words. This is all about you—you knowing yourself, you loving yourself, you adoring yourself, and you nourishing yourself. You, you, and you, and oh yes, you—that is who is getting ALL the attention now.

When you hear this, what are you noticing in your body? Is your gut clenching? Are you tuning out? Did you stop breathing? What emotions are being evoked for you? Are any judgments or negative self-talk trying to creep in? This is normal, and you are right on track.

As mothers, we are not used to having all (or any of) the positive attention on us. Oh, oops I forgot about that one day a year, Mother's Day, where receiving cards and flowers and a little extra attention should suffice as acknowledgment for a year's worth of physical and emotional labor. Ongoing, consistent positive regard for ourselves is new and uncomfortable, which is why I ask you to make a PACT with yourself as we explore what it is to live in alignment with your Cosmic Codes. In this context, a PACT is you having Patience, Affirmation, Compassion, and Trust in yourself and the world as you venture into living true to your rewritten Mother Code.

Patience

Another code we need to explode and rewrite is the one telling us that we are immediately supposed to know how to do something we have never done before—like mothering a child (or two or three), or starting a business (or two or three). No matter how impossible or irrational we know this is, many of us still think we are supposed to know how to do it, and there is no allowance for mistakes.

You wouldn't chastise a child for every fall before they learn to walk. No, you cheer them on through every stage, from creeping like a lizard to pushing up on their arms, scooting along the floor, to crawling, to standing, to walking with assistance, to eventually taking a first step, falling a lot, taking more steps, and doing it repeatedly until they can run. This entire process is hugely important for a soon-to-be toddler because the movements in each step are the building blocks for brain development. Just as we have patience with a child during this stage of development, we need to do the same for ourselves.

We have been going through learning to walk as a species for so long, the steps are wired in and, for the most part, happen naturally. Learning to live your Mother Code is a new phenomenon and one that is conceivable only because of evolution and the development of a frontal lobe, so we need a lot of patience. And like a baby's brain developing through all the stages, there is a growing body of literature supporting the idea that mothers learn, develop, and grow right alongside the child's development.[1] This is a powerful notion that upends the myth that the mother must be subsumed by the raising of the child.

---

1   These are some excellent examples of that research: Leap, Nicky, and Tricia Anderson. "The role of pain in normal birth and the empowerment of women." *Normal Childbirth: Evidence and Debate* 29 (2008); Prinds, Christina, Niels Christian Hvidt, Ole Mogensen, and Niels Buus. "Making existential meaning in transition to motherhood—a scoping review." *Midwifery* 30, no. 6 (2014): 733-741.

This concept of *growing up with your child* is real, and it benefits both mother and child in ways we are only beginning to realize. Research from the fields of human development, neuroscience, and applied learning argues that the interdependence of mother and child is often overlooked as a critical learning node for childhood development. A child's awareness of the complex ways people interact and influence one another is stunted by a model of motherhood in which happiness and nurturing are not considered a priority for mother *and* child.

Too often I see mothers who consider it noble and their duty to give their child what they didn't have. There is nothing wrong with wanting to provide our children with the best conditions for their development, but it eclipses the unconscious desire to still have our unmet needs fulfilled. We somehow assume that giving it all to them will automatically erase the lacking in our childhood. From my experience, that's not how it works. We cannot bypass our healing by helping others. If you want to heal your wounds, instead of doing it through your child, note what you are adamant about giving your children and tag it as unfinished business to work on in your own coaching or therapy.

Fortunately, your Cosmic Codes invite you to give yourself what you didn't get as you raise your child. You didn't know that when you birthed a child, you would raise two for the price of one, and that second one is you! This takes some practice, but imagine you are telling your infant how beautiful and precious they are. Easy peasy, right? Then, imagine you are also holding yourself— like twins—and that same loving energy is flowing into tiny you. Through this practice it makes real the saying, "It is never too late to have a happy childhood!"

I also encourage you to be in dialogue with your infant and children. Talk about how you are on the journey together, learning and growing and you have every intention to do your best, but you will make mistakes. This isn't an excuse for wrongdoing but an acknowledgment that mistakes will be made, and you will keep working on them.

I didn't catch on to this until my kids were a little older, but when I did, it helped us repair the inevitable attachment breaches.[2] Rather than throw out a hollow "I'm sorry" when I snapped at one of them or send a rain of negative self-talk down on myself at what a bad mother I am, I would recognize that they were getting an emotional charge that wasn't about *them*—it was often about something else that happened during the day unrelated to them. Sure, they were engaging in annoying or disruptive behavior, but my reaction was at a ten when it warranted a two. So, we would have a do-over where we would replay the interaction with an appropriate level response.

One time, when my youngest daughter, Hannah, was in second grade I came into her room with a big charge, ranting at her about something, I don't even remember what.

She looked at me and said, "Mommy, do you need a coaching session?" This stopped me in my tracks.

Instead of placating her, I surrendered to the invitation and said, "Yes, I think I do!"

To which she patted the spot next to her and said, "Ok, sit down. Now, tell me about your day."

What a gift she gave me, but also that I gave her by taking her seriously and allowing us both to repair.

I hope you see that patience isn't about waiting around for things to happen; it is about engaging in the process of your becoming with gentleness. I will also continue to acknowledge that learning new things and engaging in new practices is stressful! This is a long game endeavor and while celebrating little victories along the way, there are no quick fixes.

---

2 The blog Take Root Therapy, run by a group of counselors out of Los Angeles, provides a good overview of attachment theory here: https://www.losangelesmftherapist.com/post/why-does-this-keep-happening-to-me-how-our-attachment-styles-can-impact-our-relationships/.

Learning to tend to yourself in the moment as you learn to tend to your child is the game.

Affirmation

I am a big fan of positive self-talk. I know affirmations can get rote and, worse, toxic, but when we engage with them intentionally, they have the power to shift a fixed or negative mindset back to a growth-based, positive one. And if there is a time in our lives when we need it the most, it is during motherhood. Motherhood and mothering is a mostly thankless job, so if you are looking outside of yourself for affirmation, you will find it sorely lacking. This is why self-affirmation is so important and even more sustaining than receiving it externally.

While this concept made sense cognitively, I was continuously looking outside of myself for validation. As someone who depended on her mother's affirmation and direction in life, I had a strong *external locus of control.* This took me a lot of growth work to shift.

This powerful concept is part of the psychological theory of locus of control, which was developed by Julian Rotter in the 1950s.[3] It is a spectrum that ranges from internal to external wherein an individual's belief regarding the extent to which they can control events in their lives is managed. Those with an internal locus of control believe that their actions and decisions significantly influence outcomes, both positive and negative. You feel empowered to shape your destiny, viewing challenges as opportunities for growth and learning. This mindset fosters a sense of personal responsibility and agency, leading to proactive problem-solving and a greater sense of control over your life. With a strong internal locus of control, you usually exhibit higher levels of resilience, and overall well-being as you navigate the complexities of motherhood.

---

3 Here is *Psychology Today*'s explanation of the locus of control: https://www.psychologyto-day.com/us/basics/locus-of-control.

But with an external locus of control, you attribute the outcomes in your life primarily to external factors such as luck, fate, or other people's actions. You feel less in control of your destiny and may perceive yourself as a victim of circumstance. This mindset can lead to feelings of helplessness, passivity, and dependency, as you believe that your efforts are unlikely to make a significant difference. Consequently, those with an external locus of control may struggle to affirm themselves, take initiative, cope with challenges, and achieve their goals because they perceive themselves as being at the mercy of external forces.

My first authentic experience of self-affirmation occurred many years into my growth work when I was in Angkor Wat, a Hindu-Buddhist temple complex in Cambodia. We had greeted the sunrise with a powerful meditation, after which we set out to individually explore the temple on our own in silence. At one point I was filled with a sense of peace and well-being like I had never experienced. Rather than stay with myself and my experience, my mind quickly went to how I would share this with the group, particularly the leaders, who I was hoping would validate me for it.

But this time, I caught myself in the behavior, and when I opened my eyes, I looked across the small body of water and saw *myself* standing at the water's edge. This "other me" was waving, jumping up and down, and celebrating my experience. It felt so real, and it felt wonderful.

Giving myself affirmation actually felt better than getting it from anyone else! And for the first time, I knew I could share it with the group like I had planned, and the affirmation would be nice, but it would be icing on the cake, and I didn't need it to validate what happened. Having this experience as a touchstone helped me then to start a practice of self-affirmation and building a strong internal locus of control.

Shifting from an external locus of control to an internal locus of control as a mother involves a conscious effort to recognize and embrace your ability to influence outcomes in your life and your family's well-being. You can start by acknowledging your achievements and the role you play in your successes, no matter how small they may seem. When you accomplish something, like successfully soothing your infant or managing a busy day (or hour!) effectively, take a moment to reflect on the skills and actions you employed to make it happen. Set realistic goals and actively work toward them, recognizing that your efforts are the driving force behind reaching these goals.

When challenges arise, instead of attributing them to bad luck or external forces, consider what you can learn from the situation and how you can adapt your approach in the future. By consistently reinforcing and affirming the belief that you have the power to influence your circumstances, you can gradually shift toward a more internal locus of control, leading to greater empowerment and fulfillment in your role as a mother.

This is all about celebrating yourself! It doesn't mean depriving yourself of external affirmation; rather, it is about putting it in perspective and adjusting the value and weight you give the two. It also includes acknowledging challenges and affirming the painful and difficult aspects and experiences of your mothering journey.

And let's not forget how challenging it can be to receive affirmation and compliments when given! Stop minimizing or waving off compliments! Say, thank you. Then shut up and let it sink in. Research shows we need to savor an affirmation given to us for at least five seconds, but even better to give it 15 or 20 seconds to gain the full benefit. Savor away!! Be patient as you let the goodness absorb into you like water into a dry sponge.

Compassion

There is never a more important time to start living the adage of filling your cup before you fill others than when having compassion for yourself. It has always bothered me that so much of what we read about compassion or when we hear people speak of it, it is all about giving it to someone else. Mind you, the concept of compassion is a beautiful thing—loving-kindness shared with another—but in our mother culture, this is also a trap based on the code that dictates you are to give to your children and spouse at the exclusion of yourself. It is my experience that the opposite is true, and compassion must first be experienced and practiced within ourselves before we can give it away. Your Mother Code is a compelling and beautiful vision, and it may even include compassion, but I want to be extra sure you are prioritizing yourself.

It also calls us to receive compassion when given to us. Like I shared about affirmation, for most of us, our self-compassion muscle is weak, and we need to strengthen it. We may mistakenly read compassion as pity, which can cause us to reject it. There is also the code admonishing us for needing it because we are trained to believe that if we were strong enough, we could handle things without this sappy compassion thing. It can feel so against our norm that compassion can even come across as someone telling us we are mothering wrong or badly.

To encompass the power inherent in compassion, let's clarify the differences between sympathy and empathy. Sympathy is when you *understand* a person's situation or distress; empathy is when we attune and can *feel* another's emotions along with them; and compassion is unlike either of the two as it encompasses a *desire* to relieve someone of their suffering. An empath can absorb someone's pain to an almost extreme level, but most women who mother will say they feel their children's pain and discomfort, as well as joy, acutely when their children experience it. With empathy, the same parts of our brain light up and react as the person we are empathizing with, mirroring their experience.

(This is also why giving yourself what you are giving your children works!)

Compassion is different because it flows from our desire to give love. You understand a person's situation because you have been through something similar, but instead of taking on their emotions as your own, you act as an objective person who cares. It's easier said than done, but that is the goal.

It's natural to feel overwhelmed, anxious, and sometimes even inadequate on your mothering journey. This is where self-compassion, as researched and brought to the mainstream by Dr. Kristin Neff, can make a significant difference in your experience. By practicing self-compassion, you can transform the way you relate to yourself during these demanding times. When you encounter moments of self-doubt or frustration, the game is to offer yourself the same kindness and understanding you would give a close friend. This will help you build emotional resilience, making it easier to cope with the ups and downs of motherhood. It can also reduce feelings of anxiety and depression, helping you to maintain a more balanced and positive outlook.

As a new mother, you will probably experience a wide range of intense feelings, from joy and love to fear, frustration, and sadness. Self-compassion involves recognizing these emotions with neutrality. By being kind to yourself, you can create a safe space to process these feelings. For example, instead of criticizing yourself for feeling overwhelmed or inadequate, you can acknowledge that emotions are natural and understandable given the challenges of motherhood. This approach helps to reduce the intensity of negative emotions and prevents them from escalating.

Trust

Sometimes, even with all the research, discernment, and gut feelings you bring to the table, living in accordance with your Mother Code will still feel like taking a leap of faith. To step into the unknown of motherhood takes tremendous courage. Trusting that things will work out even when you don't have all the answers or guarantees is valiant and brave.

Trust is the ultimate vulnerability. When you choose to surrender and put your trust in someone, you expose yourself to the possibility of being let down, deceived, or hurt. The fear of betrayal or disappointment is real, and it makes trust a vulnerable act, as it requires you to put faith in others' intentions and actions. Trusting someone else means relinquishing a degree of control over a situation, which can be challenging in the throes of new motherhood. This is because it involves giving up the security that comes from managing or predicting outcomes yourself. Trusting also involves opening yourself up emotionally and sharing thoughts, feelings, or resources. This exposure adds to the vulnerability because it can lead to emotional pain if the trust is broken.

Experiences of broken trust can heighten your sense of vulnerability. If you have been hurt or betrayed before, it becomes more challenging to trust again, as the memory of past pain influences your willingness to be vulnerable. But, despite these vulnerabilities, trust is essential in fulfilling our yearnings for meaningful relationships and deep connections and creating a sense of community and belonging.

You can put a stake in the ground and decide to live from a trusting place and then know you will need to nurture and cultivate it. I had the pleasure of working with the meditation master, davidji, and can attest that his nickname, the "Velvet Voice of Stillness," is spot on. At the time of our meeting, I was not familiar with his work, but after a few days of sunrise meditations, I felt the deep impact of the healing space he created. It was cosmic timing for me because I was getting more and more clear that I needed to leave the organization I had been a part of for 32 years. I was taking a leap of faith, and davidji's meditation "Manifest More Trust in Your Life (Let Go of FEAR)"4 was a beautiful affirmation I was on the right path.

Finding Your Team

Understanding the role of the Mother Code in your life and learning how to take control and rewrite it is an exercise in the discernment of the highest order. What you are undertaking is no less than a realignment of the way you perceive and live in the world. It is also a change in how you see yourself and how you see others.

You are never alone. We established this cosmic reality in the previous chapter. You already have people around you who will be open to your vision; you also have people around you who will reject it and will try to keep you tethered to the old Mother Code in the name of helping you. Distinguishing between people who will lift you up and support your growth and those who will be an obstacle is both critical and doable.

As you grow into your Mother Code and live it, some people in your circle may not fit anymore. This is challenging but important to recognize. You need people who will support you authentically in the vision you have for yourself. You need people who will tell you the truth when you are off track and cheer you on when doing well!

Human Team

Women are given mixed messages when developing woman-to-woman relationships. The cultural rules dictate we should be nice to one another and not hurt each other's feelings. This leads us to not being truthful with one another. Men are generally given more permission to be openly competitive and direct with their criticism. We are not, so we can become passive-aggressive, judgmental, and destructive. Also, as I mentioned earlier, our insecurity in trying to live any of the impossible codes pits us against each other,

---

4 You can hear my conversation with davidji on the Rewrite the Mother Code with Gertrude Lyons, Ep 88: Using Meditation to Find Balance and Purpose in Your Life with davidji.

making us judge one another as inadequate so we can feel better about ourselves.

The hardest but most important early challenges you will face are attracting the right people around you and building boundaries to protect yourself from people who might not align with your desired experience. Think about all of the obstacles to your growth that the Mother Code has instilled in you, and push through. This growth will define the rest of your life. It is worth every bit of effort it takes. It is your birthright.

A challenge that many women I work with face as they begin to develop a practice of self-care is the choice between serving oneself and serving others. That is a false choice! Again, look at any system in nature, and you will find that improving any part of the system improves the whole. Many women I have known over the years in unhealthy relationships were told that they were being selfish when they asserted their right to take care of themselves. This is a tool of manipulation that works on people who consider taking care of others an important value.

The work we are doing together now is both/and work. You don't have to choose between the people you care about and yourself. Healing yourself *is healing those you love, too*! The opposite is true too: When those around you begin to focus on personal development, this lifts you up.

This is not just true of family and close friends. When society is operating properly, we strengthen the *koinonia*, the civic collective, with every step we take toward strengthening ourselves. As you grow within your own rewritten Mother Code, you will find yourself with women walking very similar paths. To make your growth work even stronger, lift these women up and support their journeys. What we are all doing collectively is nothing less than healing the world.

Through this work, we have the potential to empower each other and become **one team**. In doing so, we are drawing other women into the safe space we've created. They, too, will be changed for the better if they can see what is woven into the sisterhood we are collectively offering. Together, we can all rewrite our Mother Codes and help each other at the same time. The deeper your understanding of how intimately connected your health and the health of women, people, and sentience everywhere is, the more you can draw from the cosmic well for your sustenance.

As you get your mom community together, I want to remind you that this is not a mothers-only call. There are lots of other people struggling with the aspects of their lives influenced by their own Mother Code. We know that women who are childfree by choice or who cannot have children are as deeply entangled in the Mother Code as those of us who have birthed babies. And a vast world of people can also benefit from rewriting their own Mother Codes. This is a universal phenomenon with special coding for mothers but by no means excluding anyone else.

And all of us—men, women, mothers, and any other category you care to add—comprise a vast network of people who will be knitted closer together if we join our energies in rewriting the Mother Code.

Spiritual Team

Tapping into the cosmic truths of the Mother Code calls you to look beyond the physical to consider that other manifestations can fortify you and guide you in this process. What a lovely surprise to find out how full the universe is of encouragement and support.

You don't have to believe in spirits, goddesses, or angels to continue along this path. I will strongly encourage you to withhold judgment of those who carry these beliefs, however. We have been acculturated to believe there is only one way to see the universe. This worldview includes the Mother Code that has held us back for so long. An inclusive perspective is a cosmic perspective. If you dig into philosophy, physics, psychology, neuroscience, and the arts (notice I am not mentioning religion), you will discover that the greatest minds and most insightful visionaries see the world as a "yes/and" place. From this perspective, there is room for all viewpoints. This is the matricentric way.

I was nine years old when my grandmother passed. I have mentioned before that her love for my grandfather and his for her—and the love they had for me as a child—was my model of healthy relationships. I relied on her. She was a rock. She was a source of limitless love.

The first time I can recall asking for support from someone beyond the physical realm was when I reached out to my deceased grandmother. During a difficult and overwhelming time, I invoked her spirit and presence. It happened as if by instinct, as if the bond had never faded, and I listened to the quiet voice inside me telling me she was still with me. Shortly after that invocation, I saw her in my dreams more and more. Eventually, I started actually feeling her holding me. It was a huge comfort. After that experience began, I spoke to her during meditation.

You will find as you rewrite your Mother Code you are peeling away many myths and limiting beliefs. Connecting with the dead is no exception. We are taught that there is only a physical world, yet when you read and listen to physicists, you discover there isn't even a truly physical world. When you get to the smallest levels of existence, everything includes waves.

Millions of people report seeing apparitions of Mary, including adults and children. Often, people report she is speaking directly to them. She often talks to people about how much she loves us, but she also expresses concern, concern for our spiritual, physical, and emotional well-being and for the state of the planet. I have not had an apparition experience, but I have felt her presence strongly.[5]

These beautiful Mary experiences occurred at Our Lady of Lourdes in France, at a shrine in the mountains of Eastern Spain in the regions of Catalonia, and at Our Lady of Fatima in Portugal. When I first felt her presence, she was very much the traditional image we associate with Mary, the feminine, loving mother, what a novelist would call a flat character. Over time, her full depth, complexity, and power became discernible. This was a gradual and mutual revelation: She was slowly revealing herself to me in sync with my ability to comprehend what I was feeling. She now comes as a representation that across time, women have revered and honored different aspects of the divine feminine.

In my experience, she is not a single, static object, creature, or goddess. I am not describing old goddesses vanquished by the Christian God or any other such fantasy novel ideas. These are cosmic presences that are beyond identity or limited forms. They are as much a part of us as they are part of the unseen they inhabit. They are simultaneously many—infinitely many—and one.

You can keep your idea of a single creator spirit and still see manifestations of various aspects of that force. These ideas do not compete. They only compete in a worldview that demands only one deity should exist, which is a limited perspective and one that will also stamp out the idea that you can create your future, that you can rewrite your Mother Code.

---

5   The literature on Mary is endless and spans millennia. Two favorites of mine are: Strand, Clark, and Perdita Finn. *The Way of the Rose: The Radical Path of the Divine Feminine Hidden in the Rosary*. Random House, 2019; and Strand, Sophie. *The Madonna Secret*. Bear and Co., 2023. I was able to talk with both of these amazing women on my podcast, Rewrite the Mother Code with Gertrude Lyons, Ep 84: *Navigating the Way of the Rose with Clark Strand and Perdita Finn.*

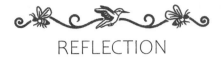

REFLECTION

Give yourself space to name and voice all the doubts, fears, judgments, and reactivity that have arisen in this or earlier chapters. Yours may range from being blissed out by having a spiritual experience to tearing out the pages and throwing them in the trash or anywhere on this continuum. But I promise you, whether you are in touch with them or not, your feelings are part of the journey of surrendering into the life that is a womb and a crucible.

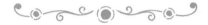

When modern archaeologists try to explain the remains of the Neolithic era, that long period of relative peace in which mass war and metal weapons did not exist, there is a totem that gets quickly characterized as a goddess. She appears in every site from the era. She comes in many shapes and sizes, sometimes thin with sharp features and sometimes physically robust, with a large belly and large breasts. Male archeologists often lump her into the general category of "fertility goddesses" due to their lack of feminine experience or creativity to think beyond a culture where a woman's only prayer would be to conceive a child. These were objects of empowerment and reflection, offering support and guidance in the innumerable desires of a woman.

We call the old gods and goddesses by those deific terms because we don't know what else to say. What I would say based on my experience of the divine feminine is that every woman is the goddess, and no one person or deity is Goddess. Divinity is in each of us. Unity is the manifestation of all of us.

Rewriting the Mother Code is like writing your own prayer to yourself, a codex of self-esteem, a bridge to your portal to the cosmos. You don't have to see apparitions or hear spirits to connect to the universal. It is already within you. But I highly encourage you to remain open to whatever might happen once you open the doors to perception.

A series of small steps carried out with intention and dedication leads to transformation. Expecting challenges and setbacks as a matter of course is a mindset well worth fostering. In making a PACT with yourself, you can tend to yourself in the most nurturing ways and heal old wounds that get pricked when you come up against opposition.

You are capable of so much more than you can imagine, and I want everything for you that you can possibly achieve. Please believe that. But also know that I am celebrating every small victory right along with you. Whatever you can do in pursuit of your own Mother Code is worthwhile effort and time well spent.

There is more to the cosmos than our five senses reveal to us. See with your intuition. See with your heart. Entire worlds, universes, planes of existence are there, awaiting your arrival. We are on an adventure both of cosmic proportions and micro-moments, which are the same.

And all of it matters!

Chapter 9
Birth Is Eternal

Back in the day of kings and knights, they would use a *standard* during the battle. It was a banner, generally designed and stitched by the hands of women, on a pole held high so everyone on the field of battle could orient to it. In the chaos of battle, it guided them physically, emotionally, and spiritually. The design or visual held significance and meaning for the region, reminding them what they were fighting for and why they were putting their lives at risk.

We see the powerful potential of a banner in the Arthurian legends. I am especially drawn to the part the women in King Arthur's universe played in this—particularly his half-sister, Morgaine, and his wife, Guinevere. I was struck by the impact of the women and the influence of Christianity, claiming the minds and hearts of people who had honored the Goddess in equal measure to God. This was a devastating turning point in history where intuition, healing arts, and sacred rituals and rites that honored the seasons were not only frowned upon but they were also considered evil works of the devil. Sound familiar?

Tragically, it was Arthur's wife Guinevere who, having bought into the new order, convinced Arthur to put down the dragon banner, break his sworn allegiance to mystical Avalon, and carry into an upcoming battle a banner she had made with a cross boldly displayed. This was an affront to the old ones, and while some put down their swords and would not follow Arthur, most joined the new standard out of fear of being unprotected. Arthur proved victorious. Did this mean that the Christian god won this battle for them? That is what Guinevere and others professed, and it wielded a lot of leverage in shifting religious and cultural belief systems.

All this to say, a standard holds our beliefs, our dreams, our wishes, and our values, and that is powerful magic. Guinevere knew this and exploited Arthur's love for her (a misuse of feminine power), using it to her advantage. While she felt righteous in doing so, the irony is she was using the same magic she was purportedly trying to suppress. She cast a spell on her husband and the people he was leading. Everyone followed suit after that because they won the battle, so it seemed to have worked. When you look deeper at Guinevere, as she is often depicted, she was a woman without a solid sense of self. She was scared to leave her castle as a little girl. The thick stone walls gave her a sense of safety and control which is why it was easy for her to gravitate to this new religion. It, too, had rigid walls where she was safe from the mysteries found in the feminine unknown.

That she managed to wander into the elusive Avalon where she met Lancelot and Morgaine for the first time could only mean she connected with the energy of the place. I imagine it was disconcerting and confusing for her to have access to the power of the feminine only to hear the propaganda that the women of Avalon were evil sorceresses. So, she chose to shut that part of herself down.

Morgaine, tagged to be the next high priestess of Avalon, ran away from this place she loved dearly because she could not reconcile the shame she felt from playing the part of the goddess at Beltane. During this rite, she unknowingly had sex with her half-brother, Arthur, and conceived a child. Suddenly lost and unsure, she wandered into the land of the fairies for what she thought was a few weeks but turned out to be four years. During that time, her mother died, Arthur had secured peace in the kingdom, and Guinevere had convinced Arthur to put down the Pendragon flag. Morgaine tried to get back into Avalon, but her way was blocked, so she went to Camelot.

While she didn't adopt the ways of Christianity, she cast aside her place in line to be the next Priestess of Avalon. Morgaine let her wisdom and hard-earned connection with the "Sight" (intuitive or psychic abilities) recede to the far background.[1]

It was only in this writing I first saw myself and my feminine journey reflected in these two women! If you recall in my story, I, too, left organized religion and reawakened my intuitive power as a woman, only to later walk away and return to the safety of the masculine in a controlling work environment. Also, like Morgaine, I didn't forsake or demonize the power of the feminine as starkly as Guinevere, but maybe worse because I pretended to be a part of a paradigm that never felt like home and slowly let the intuitive parts of me go underground.

I also claim the Guinevere in me. I was that scared little girl that felt safest in my home. I left the unruly public high school of my hometown for a Catholic, all-girls, boarding school. I was tall, blonde, pretty, and had been treated like a dress-up doll by my mother, so I mistakenly thought that was where my value lied. I was not encouraged to think for myself and when I

---

1 This mythology is so deeply embedded in Western culture that there are myriad sources with a variety of perspectives to draw upon to learn about the women of the Arthurian legend. A sympathetic telling of Morgaine's story can be found at https://theconversation.com/morgan-le-fay-how-arthurian-legend-turned-a-powerful-woman-from-healer-to-villain-109928. An interesting compilation of women's interpretations of the legend is listed at https://d.lib.rochester.edu/camelot/text/marsh-women-of-the-arthurian-legend.

found myself queen to "King Richard" I assumed my value was to bring his children into the world. I shrunk myself so as not to risk losing the security of home and a comfortable life. It didn't matter that this line of thinking did not make rational sense as my husband had shown he could withstand my appetite to push the boundaries of the status quo. I believe that this irrational fear was something much older, from generations past, that was playing out in this lifetime.

Finding my reflection in these mythic women is powerful and humbling. Through time and self-reflection, I can see the mythic journey of my moments in motherhood. Like so many mythic quests, there is usually an elder or sage or faery queen guiding the way, and foretelling how the journey will be filled with challenges. Sometimes there are specific directives—slay the dragon, obtain the fleece from the golden lamb or a scale from a dragon... you know the drill. Other times they offer words of warning—beware of the sirens in the sea, or the faery in the forest who will promise safe haven, etc.

Inevitably, even with these cautions, the quester finds themselves in all sorts of perilous pickles of one kind or another. But the true quest is accumulating wisdom, strengthening muscles, riding the waves of doubt and despair, and finding inner and outer fortitude and resilience not possessed before.

So much of what emerges in your Cosmic Codes is written into myths and legends. You are so drawn to these stories because they offer a treasure trove of possibility for your return to who you are. When you can see yourself in the women of these legends you can strengthen your allegiance to your rewritten Mother Codes and from there lift off into cosmic consciousness as you engage in the ecstatic journey of continuously birthing yourself. This is when you start living a new reality and seasons of mothering morph into moments of cosmic mothering!

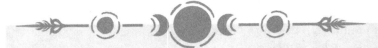

WOMB OPENING RITUAL

With the new reality that your womb is so much more than a group of organs making a baby grow inside of you, I offer this meditation. Use it to honor and deepen your relationship with the cosmic energy and vastness of the womb space of creation that resides in all of us.

Begin by bringing your hands together in front of you. Touch the tips of your thumbs together, and then touch the tips of your index fingers together, forming a triangle with your hands. This triangle is a symbol of creation, representing the sacred energy of your womb (or for men, the Sacral Chakra).

Gently place this triangle of your hands over your womb area—just below your navel. Feel the warmth of your hands connecting with this powerful center of your body. For men, place the triangle over your Sacral Chakra, just below the belly button. Let your hands rest here, creating a direct connection to your creative and life-giving energy.

With your hands resting on your womb, focus on the energy within this space. As you connect with this light, speak aloud or in your mind:

"I open my womb—I conceive, I create, I birth."

Feel the power of these words resonating within you. You may say them once, letting the energy expand with each word, or repeat them as a chant, letting the rhythm and vibration build within your womb. Each repetition strengthens your connection to your creative power and

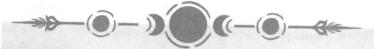

your ability to bring forth new life, ideas, and expressions.

As you continue to repeat the words, imagine your womb opening like a flower, petals unfurling to receive and give life. Let this energy fill your entire body, flowing from your womb out into the world, connecting you to the infinite potential of the universe. Feel the strength, creativity, and life force that resides within you, fully awakened and ready to manifest.

When you feel complete, let the chant gently fade, returning to the silence within.

Take a few more deep breaths, feeling the energy of your womb still vibrating, alive with possibility.

This meditation is designed to connect deeply with your creative and life-giving energy, empowering you to bring forth new life, ideas, and expressions from the sacred space of your womb. It can be practiced whenever you feel the need to activate and honor your creative power.

Moments of Cosmic Motherhood

"It took two years to conceive Morgan, I think we should get started now if we want a three-year age gap between them," I said to my husband in February of 1998.

He agreed.

At this moment, Rich and I were engaging in some intense growth work. To promote greater honesty and intimacy, we were encountering each other with unfiltered emotional expression.

It was vulnerable, freeing, and exhilarating—and scary to be honest. It was from this raw open space we opened the doors to conceiving our second child.

I was pregnant immediately!

So much for time to plan and prepare like we had our first. This soul saw the window crack open and flew right in! I had always wanted to have the experience I'd read about where the woman feels the spark of conception at the moment of intercourse. This did not happen for me. But what happened was its own version of magic.

When Morgan was 18 months old, we went on a vacation to Santa Fe, New Mexico. Everything about this trip felt heightened— the moon was huge; the spiritual sites we visited were crackling with energy; and I was notably out of breath while we were hiking in Chaco Canyon. During this hike, where the remains of a massive ceremonial complex covered in celestial patterns remains a mystery, we came upon ancient petroglyphs. Morgan almost launched herself out of the backpack carrier to touch the spiral carved into the stone. She slowly traced it with her finger. We were all transfixed.

Was it simply toddler curiosity or was she connecting and communicating with the ancient peoples who made these carvings? As I recall the sensations in my body at that moment, it was the latter.

That same night I drew a warm bath. Under the glow of the moon, I spontaneously welcomed the soul that had arrived in my womb. It was a blessed and sacred moment. When I emerged from the water, I shared the unconfirmed news with Rich. After returning to Chicago, we created a little ceremony to verify what I knew to be true with a pregnancy test. Tears of joy rolled down both of our cheeks.

We caught ourselves up with the exercises in *The Conception Mandala*, and while this soul had already made their way in, we sent a formal invitation, set our wishes and desires, and created a mandala.

When we found out the due date was December 21st, I was delighted that she might be born on the Winter Solstice. Rather than be upset it was during the holidays, I thought it was propitious to be happening during this holy time of the year. More than a few people let us know how terrible it is to have a birthday during the holidays because it would forever be eclipsed by the hubbub of celebrating Christmas. Spoken as an order that I recognized as a Mother Code, I continued to be delighted in welcoming a child at this auspicious time.

I had labor pains on the solstice, but they came and went. I was disappointed. Christmas Eve rolled around, and the weather was unseasonably mild for Chicago, such that when I lit lanterns outside in my burgundy velvet maternity dress, I was coatless. Craving Christmas music, we popped in our neighborhood church and listened to hymns. Santa Claus came that night, the next morning we opened presents, and the three of us had a full but restful day.

Rich had given me several movies on DVD and after we put Morgan to bed, we watched two. The first was *Phenomenon*. In this film, the main character, played by John Travolta, is struck by a beam of light walking home from the bar after his birthday party. This event gives him the ability to access parts of his brain that brought about superhuman sensory perception, insight, and lightning-fast accessibility to knowledge acquisition. What was (and still is) so touching about this movie is that he accessed and honored all aspects of his heightened awareness. It equally displayed his grasp of the most complex forms of knowledge as well as his intuitive senses and connection with the energy of the earth, such that he could predict an earthquake before it happened.

Despite it getting late, we went ahead with the second movie, which was *Contact*. In the film, a little girl, Ellie, asks her dad if he believes there are people on other planets. He responds, "I don't know, Sparks (her nickname). But I guess I'd say if it is just us… seems like an awful waste of space." Her father passes away shortly after this, and we next see Ellie as an adult astrophysicist researcher (played by Jodie Foster) dedicating her life to making contact with life on other planets. I won't share any more specifics of what unfolds for Ellie, but it exemplifies our continued struggle to bring scientific findings in harmony with the truth of our experience. It feels appropriate to add here that throughout this pregnancy, as with Morgan's, I saw a holistic, kinesiologist practitioner. During one of our visits, I asked if there was anything about their cosmic origins or past lives he could sense. He said that Morgan was an old soul who had lived many lifetimes here on earth, but that the baby I carried was a star child and this would be their first Earth experience. So, was it a coincidence that the movie we watched right before going into labor was about connecting with life on other planets, or was it a message from the cosmos? While I always held it as a beautiful portent and blessing, it was not until writing this and going back to read pertinent lines from the movie that I saw how clear and obvious the message was.

We wrapped up our double feature at 1:00 am, and as I crawled into bed I felt a twinge of a contraction. I wrote it off, but I thought I better get to sleep because if this time it's for real I will need my rest. I told Rich I was feeling intermittent pangs, and we both went to sleep. I woke up at 4:00 am and the contractions were stronger, but there were gaps, and since my first birth evolved over 26 hours from the first contraction, I thought it best to get more rest. When I woke at 7:00 am, I knew my labor was progressing. I called our midwife.

"Why haven't you called me sooner!?" were the first words out of Kate's mouth when she heard my voice. Midwives don't need to see you to know where you are in your labor. I never had an internal exam through the whole birth process. Why poke around in there unless you need to?

Kate said she would be over immediately.

Hearing her urgency kicked things into high gear for me. I knew I was in full-blown labor. I was shaking with what felt like chills, but it was the energy of birth coursing through my body. We tried calling our friends Jenn and Scott to be with Morgan while I gave birth. This was before reliable cell phone service, and they were in a place without a signal, and we didn't have a landline number for them. So, our midwife contacted a doula friend who would come over on short notice the day after Christmas.

Rich, also thinking we had a long day ahead of us, was in the shower when our first midwife arrived. He quickly dressed, and just by looking at me, Kate said I was going to have this baby this morning. It was 8:00 am.

"What? This doesn't make sense. Don't I have all day and possibly into the night?" I asked between intense contractions where I gripped Rich's arm so tight I thought I would break it.

Kate and Rich left the bathroom, where I was kneeling next to the tub, shivering and gripping the edge as contractions came. When they went to gather supplies, it was just Morgan and me together in the space when another contraction came. I cried out in pain. I remember yelling "Mama" and being surprised I would invoke the help of my mother at this time.

During the next contraction, Morgan stood next to me and said, "You can do it, Mommy, keep going!" Then she offered me her little two-year-old arm to grab like she had seen Rich do for me.

Between contractions I thanked her for her encouragement but told her I would break her arm if I grabbed it. The next contraction came, and it was a strong one. Morgan silently slipped behind me, placed her little hands on my hips and swayed them gently but firmly back and forth. My pain was instantly alleviated. Unlike my arm holding, no one had modeled this for her.

Where did this wisdom come from? How did she know to do this? I get teary and full of goosebumps whenever I share this experience because I know there are no rational answers.

Before I could give any more thought to the miracle that just happened, Rich and our midwives Kate and Mary entered the bathroom. Morgan, still in her Santa pajamas, lingered nearby. After observing my next contraction, Mary and Kate said, "You are going to have this baby in the next half-hour." It was 9:00. Soon after, they said I would have her in the next four pushes. Right as she crowned, Morgan stepped out of the room. Our new baby girl entered the world at 9:35 am—precisely the time they said she would—after four pushes. Morgan came back in as soon as her new sister was in my arms.

Rivers of energy coursed through my body. I held this new miracle in my arms as Mary peeled a layer of a filmy substance from her face. While we waited for the umbilical cord to stop pulsing, they explained that she had been born in her bag of water and it didn't break until she crowned (when the head begins to emerge from the birth canal). The filmy substance was her bag of water. Midwives refer to this as being born in the caul, or under the veil, and it was an auspicious, holy, and rare occurrence.

Once the umbilical cord stopped pulsing with life and Rich cut the cord, I soon delivered the placenta. Mary and Kate held it up and laughed. They said, "Look at this, your placenta is heart shaped! At this point we would expect nothing less!"

This is cosmic birthing!

Yes, there was intense pain, even more than normal because a baby being born in their bag of water means that while she had some extra buoyancy and cushion, I had extra pressure as she come through the birth canal. Amid this pain I was also conscious of all the intense sensations I was having—shivers of energy and aliveness, the heat of Morgan's touch, the sounds of my voice. I sought the protection and support of the Divine Mother by invoking Her name.

I was present to my toddler daughter channeling midwifery and lifting the pain during an intense contraction. I watched as they pulled the veil from my newborn daughter's head. I laughed with joy as our midwives held up the heart-shaped placenta. It was all there in the exquisite alchemy of birth.

I was all there!

We took a week to find the right name for this new being. The ones we picked out just didn't seem to fit her. (Another bonus of a home birth is the flexibility of turning in official documents.) When we came upon Hannah, it felt right. We didn't make it official until we checked the numerology and the origins of the name meaning grace or favor. We were graced and favored with miracles as she came into the world!

The Joy of the Cosmos

You planted yourself in your mother's womb. You get to choose how you want your seed to flourish and grow. Now that you have broken the spell and reawakened yourself to reality, you get to play! Here is a little-known secret—cosmic motherhood is fun! When we understand that Universe wants the best for us and wants us to learn and grow and make mistakes and try again and play. Play with this life. Play with the journey of your creation. When I revisit the experience of the births of my daughters, I am filled with awe and wonder. I am bursting with gratitude as well as tremendous excitement, fear, pain, and ecstatic revelation that life is a playground where the birthing of my daughters will forever be a landmark moment in my life.

When I uncovered the false duality of pleasure and pain, the connection I felt to the cosmos and my own divinity, and the affirmation of my deeply intuitive choice (against the voices of so many people) to deliver them at home—I fully embodied my rewritten Mother Code. All of it drives me to do what I do today. There is an experience waiting for every mother through birthing with no equivalent in the world. Our being pressured—even bullied and compelled—to abandon this in preference to a numbed version of our miraculous selves through a deceptively enticing drug-induced stupor would be a dystopian plot line if it weren't an everyday reality all over the planet.

You have a right to experience the delivery of your child! What we learn about our limitless potential during labor and birth is so threatening to the social order that we are over-medicated even where some pain management is justified to minimize its power. You have a potential inside of you that some would love to hide from you forever, and the Mother Code is intended to do just that.

This is why we must rewrite it, because mothering was never meant to be an assembly line event. Every birth is unique. Every mother is unique. You are a scintillating spark lofted into the cosmos in a unique way, and when you conceive, you engage in the wondrous act of creation. From that moment through delivery, a silver thread connects you to the birth of stars and the formation of galaxies. You are literally part of a cosmic dance which animates all things. How incredible you are!

Experience the awesome power of your body and that relationship to the universe. I want your unique version of what I experienced for you and mothers everywhere. I know without a doubt that it is available to all of us, including women after the birth of your children. None of this experience is erased, only buried under an oppressive framework that degrades our identities and robs us of our potential. All your possibility as a mother is tied to an intimacy with the cosmic law of creation that goes beyond medical procedures and technological tools.

Every birth is an opening to a cosmic gateway, and this miracle takes place every quarter of a second all over the world. We in the West have been acculturated to believe that miracles must be rare, yet all over the world, older cultures see miracles every day. Even Europeans believed that saints and holy manifestations of the miraculous were ubiquitous a few hundred years ago. Every life deserves a miracle, and every life begins with one. Mothers are the everyday miraculous all around us.

When I reached an epiphany during my first birth, I knew without question I was a goddess. And I know that about each of you as well. When my two-and-a-half-year-old daughter channeled midwife wisdom at the birth of my second daughter, I could no longer doubt the mother energy that courses through all of us, no matter the age. We are a divine constellation, ringing the planet with our power to bring life into the world. I call upon all of us to fulfill the potential of that power, to begin to live in conscious realization of our own potential and that of all kinds of mothers everywhere—mothers who are always, everywhere, incredible.

Be the goddess you are! No matter how or what you believe, this message is for you, and this sisterhood is your home. Let us all come together in community and change ourselves, our loved ones, our neighborhoods, and our planet. The world is in desperate need of our voices.

New Motherhood

In my experience, most, if not all, women would include the words *it is hard* in a conversation about new motherhood. I mean come on, how could anyone sail through an event that is so profound and beautiful as well as completely life-altering, full of utter chaos, and constant disruption of life? Even if you have cared for children in your life, having your own experience will stir up so much so fast it is impossible to keep up, which is why you need ALL the tools and frameworks I share in this book. You need your VOICE. You need your Mother Code and the Cosmic Codes. You need your PACT. If you can invoke these in your day, you will find a space of calm in the storm. Even if you cannot recall it all perfectly, you can remember it exists and that you are having a profound experience that no amount of planning can prepare you for.

The magic in new motherhood is all about surrendering expectations of what this should look and feel like. You will probably have bouts of strong emotions. If these become so overwhelming you cannot care for your infant, seek the support of a therapist.

Also know that it is safe to have these emotions, and it is more important than ever that you let them flow.

It is also about surrendering to Yin energy. In a culture that has trained us to believe the unknown and dark forest is scary, being in this space could feel foreign. You may have the impulse to get back to normal (aka back in control) or get your body back (aka denial of what your body has been through and not celebrating it). Recognize that as part of a disempowering spell, we are under and surrender to ebbs and flows that make up the experience of new motherhood.

I will never claim I navigated this territory in the way I think is possible—a way which I have seen other women accomplish, but with my first, I maintained a sense of all the upset being fodder for my growth. With my second I wish I had reached out for more support. I thought I was supposed to know what I was doing, given it was my second child, but having an infant and a toddler put me into a tailspin. I regressed to that little Guinevere-like girl who didn't feel safe leaving the house.

Coaching women in this space has helped me heal the wound of my disappearance and have compassion for the woman I was at that time. It is so beautifully reciprocal.

Toddlers

When I think about toddler years and applying your Cosmic Codes, it is all about living the "P" in PACT—patience. You are called to slow down and enter the world of curiosity, wonder, awe, and exponential growth. We give so much of our mother energy to these little beings as they navigate the transition of complete helplessness to their first acts of independence—weaning, walking, potty training, to name a few of the big ones.

This is an ideal time to practice putting your wounded little self right next to them as you encourage, guide, and celebrate them for every movement toward their goal. You will also be triggered by their growing will and testing of boundaries. It is normal to have upset, and you will find lots of hidden treasure when you give your-self space to explore the strong feelings and reactions that come up.

My mother's desires and demands dictated my upbringing, so rather than going to the other side of the pendulum and letting them run the show, I took the advice of Alfred Adler and Rudolf Dreikurs and gave them choices. This is a simple example, but my mom laid out my clothes for me until I was in 7th grade. This kind of behavior made it difficult for me to make simple choices later in life. So, I found a balance. Rather than turn it completely over to them, I let them choose among a set of options. If what they picked was not my choice or, God forbid, the outfit didn't match, I got to tend to my desire to control and risk other mothers judging me as a bad mom. By putting myself in the mix and offering the encour-agement to choose without judgment, I was giving my daughters that which helped me heal that wound.

This applies to the big stuff and the little stuff. Pick any mo-ment in your day as a mother, and you will find places where you experience the impact of the wiring of our Mother Codes.

School Years

Early school and preteen years aren't necessarily easy, but they can offer a calm before the storm of the teenage years. You have more instances of your children wanting to be with you, being open to your support and guidance, and while there are challenges, they don't seem as big.

But this is a time to check our tendency to create drama and problems where none exist. I see this happen because of the inten-sive mothering and carpenter paradigms that dictate it is our job to do everything for our child, sculpt them into our likeness, and feel our total worth from their needing us. Reminder: they are not ours, and spoiler alert: it is not in their benefit to be so. As someone with a mother who both lived vicariously through me and, worse, tried to shield me from the inevitable pains of growing up, I know the crippling impact of these behaviors. I would not call my mom a helicopter parent, but she hovered into my business and made it clear that she knew best and following her guidance would be most beneficial. Well, it wasn't, and I have had to work hard to build, differentiate, and trust myself and my decisions.

This is an important time to develop your life outside the responsibilities of caretaking for your children and possibly your partner. Your Cosmic Codes are so important here as they orient you toward your personal development as well as meeting your deeper yearning. But most of all, they let you set the standard for what success is rather than have that dictated by family or culture.

During this development period, many parents fall into the trap of over-scheduling their children. We need to distinguish between providing nourishing learning environments and the trap of preparing them for an Ivy League college when they are six years old. This feeds the masculine paradigm of checking boxes and goal setting as the only means of value and success in our lives. Resisting it is challenging. I did not hold up well under the pressure. I let them quit ballet for soccer. I had them in scheduled activities all the time. I dropped things like creating rituals together or making sure there was plenty of space to be still with themselves. I regret some of these decisions, but I am also aware this is where I need a lot of compassion and grace for myself.

Teenagers

For many years, I held standards, imposed logical consequences when necessary, and reveled in them saying they hated me—because I knew that meant I was doing my job of instilling independence within limits. I didn't care if they liked me, and that was a gift I feel I gave them. Let's fast forward to the teen years, and I admit it was the stage I feel I didn't do as well—particularly regarding harnessing the potential for my growth and healing. I had so much unfinished business that got activated, but I avoided working on it. I blocked the light from hitting the prism, put my head down, and got through it.

When our daughter started rebelling and testing our limits, I was beside myself. What happened? Where did we go wrong? She was making choices we didn't think were healthy. Well, come to find out, there isn't a right and wrong on these matters. They are supposed to push the boundaries on their pathway to discovering themselves and deciding who they are and how they will navigate the world without us.

Again, this doesn't mean the answer is to let them do what they want. It is to get clear for ourselves what our standards are and to stick to them—even if they tell us that we've ruined their lives. It was a balance of giving them freedom where we could and then holding them accountable consistently with clear and logical consequences if they ventured outside the parameters of our boundaries.

This was an opportunity to return to our teenage years along with them. That is what I regret avoiding, and I believe that not doing this made the whole time so much harder. I know that with a little more distance and clarity around my teenage wounds and mindset, this could have been a time of considerable healing, mutual learning, and growing together.

Leaving Home

I was ready! Sometimes, I feel like a bad mom when I hear women share how sad they are to have their children leave home. I was not sad. I was so proud of them and highly valued our precious and fleeting time together. I was ready for them to go. That part of my responsibility was complete, and I was ready to move to my next phase. Being so clear about that gave them the runway to fly. If we have resistance to letting go, they will unconsciously have trouble separating, even if they move out of the house. It has helped foster a move from an adult-child relationship to an adult-adult relationship.

This does not mean we are free from Mother Codes limiting and restricting the fullness of our experience in this phase of our mothering journey. These codes may not be ever-present, but they usually come up during various transitions in our adult children's lives. This became apparent when our daughter got engaged, and I had the role of MOB—mother of the bride. This role was a source of pride and celebration and another opportunity to rewrite many Mother Codes to ultimately claim my value and heal from lifetimes of misogyny baked into this important milestone in our daughter's life.

Like so many of the mothering spaces, this one has its own flavor and set of rules and codes. There are codes about what my job was and my place in the planning and participation of common rituals. I noticed codes that harkened back to the days when women were property with no agency in the decision of who they would wed and when. I also realized early on that the choices I made at the time of my wedding regarding how much I included my mother in the planning did not reflect my daughter's experience. I was so afraid my thoughts and support were unwanted or that I would be too much it led my daughter to first think I wasn't interested in doing the planning with her.

What I worked out for myself through their engagement and wedding was threefold. First I was met with the joy and pain that came back from when I got married back in 1990. Second was confronting the anger I felt toward enacting rituals that reflected male domination and then deciding what I would do about it. And lastly, I was working my feelings around the last birthing of my daughter into the world.

All the phases of mothering a child I have shared here are births—a death to an old phase and the emergence of a new one. In each birth, there was a severing of ties. I realized that starting with my spiritual conception experience in Ireland, to Morgan's birth from my womb to all the ones along the way, I would be alone. Nobody else at the wedding could have my experience because they did not birth her. I would be completely alone. People could support me, but no one was in my body. It became crystal clear that we birth alone, and we die alone.

This helped so much because I first didn't understand why Rich couldn't relate. There is no parallel. Rich's relationship to Morgan is less complicated and more explicitly defined. This takes me back to my second area of using my Cosmic Codes as the MOB. Going for my satisfaction and claiming what I wanted was a facet of my growth that I was working on. When I looked at the wedding traditions, where the father walks her down the aisle and "gives her to the groom" and gives the toast at the reception, I had feelings. I was hurt and angry about the assumptions pervading these traditions. Morgan said she would be happy to have us both walk her down and each give a speech if that is what I wanted. I thought about it, but somehow, that wasn't meeting my yearning to bring feminine being and ritual to the event. And then, during a meditation, I got it. I was to create a bridal blessing for Morgan and all the women. Morgan was all for the idea!

What followed was two months of wakeful nights as I communed with spirit, mainly in the energy of Mary, to conceive what I called a bridal blessing, but really was a calling in of the wisdom of ancient generations of women before me. I wasn't coming up with anything new. I was breathing life back into a ritual that went underground when it wasn't safe for women to be with their intuition or expressions of joy and freedom.

The words from the Beatles song, "Let It Be," came to me. This song had deep resonance with me and my best friend, who had recently passed from lung cancer, and our husbands from the same Ireland trip. I knew right then that I had to call in the ancestors to the blessing. Jenn was my daughter's godmother. I then added another layer and asked Jenn's daughter (Rich's goddaughter) to come earlier than she planned and sing the song at the blessing. When I tell you there was not a dry eye in the house, I am not exaggerating.

I felt so divinely guided in the preparation and that day. My only regret was downplaying it and making it sound like it was just this little offering and time for the women to gather for a bit when it was so much more sacred and profound than even I thought it would be. It was so powerful a woman there asked if I would do one before her upcoming wedding. Another asked if I would do one when she conceived her first baby. Hence, a blessing sending my daughter off to her next phase of life and my offering for rites of passage blessings were born.

Were it not for my following of my initial agitation and reawakened awareness that my satisfaction mattered, none of this would have come to pass. As the matriarch, I had to hold everything and everyone's experience in my consciousness. I was vast enough to encompass everyone and everything and not leave myself behind.

When the Woman Becomes the Warrior

In Mesopotamian folklore and some Jewish mystical traditions, Adam has a partner before Eve, a woman named Lilith. Mesopotamian mythology names her as a demon, a seductress, and an agent of chaos. Jewish tradition sometimes calls her Adam's first wife but also characterizes her as a demon in other places. Christianity's long tradition of marginalizing women begins with almost total disregard for this important figure, but some scholars believe that a shadow of her remains in the extant, albeit deracinated, text.[2]

"God created man in his own image, in the image of God created he him; male and female created he them," the King James Bible tells us in Genesis chapter 1, verse 27. That scholars distinguish between the woman referenced here and Eve is the reasonable

---

2 This blog attempts to provide a balanced account of Lilith within the context of Jewish literature: https://www2.kenyon.edu/Depts/Religion/Projects/Reln91/Power/lilith.htm. An account drawing from a broader range of sources appears here: https://skhadka.sites. gettysburg.edu/Lilith/lilith-in-ancient-texts/.

consequence of her origin. Eve is not created in the same way as Adam; she is derived from him, an act of profound symbolic significance. Women owe their existence to the existence of men; men are the original created beings, and women are derivative and secondary. But what about the first woman? What about Lilith?

As in the story of all too many women in history, Lilith must be largely reconstructed rather than researched. But Jewish literature picks up where the Bible leaves off, providing a little more detail. A woman is created alongside Adam. She is his first wife—Lilith, in Hebrew. But Lilith does not see herself as secondary to Adam. She demands equality. She won't lie underneath Adam during sex. When Adam demands that she submit to him, she leaves him and the Garden of Eden. Angels are sent to retrieve her, and she refuses to return. They threaten the lives of her children, which must have numbered in the thousands, warning her they will kill 100 a day until she returns to Adam.

I can't imagine what Lilith would have done in league with the serpent at the Tree of Knowledge. It's a sure thing that she would not have been ashamed because she learned more about the world. After reflection, what seems to be a bit of errata on the margins of the pristine Christian creation story could be an apt bridge between what came before Eden and the world that it shapes the Earth into. Adam and Eve are meant to be the first man and woman, but this detail—documented, remember, even in the Bible, where God's first invention of woman is alongside man, not from his rib—seems instead to be God's first approved man and woman. The starting point of the history of the Bible coincides with the start of what scholars call the birth of civilization. This period is also the end of the age of matricentric societies during the Neolithic era, a time known for the discovery of agriculture, women-centered villages, and an absence of large-scale conflict.

Lilith seems so much like a character out of this Neolithic era that one inevitably wonders if there is some unconscious truth in these mythologies related to the transition of human culture from pre-Bronze Age, agricultural, mother-centered communities to an age that might be better described as the First Age of Metal Weapons than the Bronze Age. Lilith demands equality, finds no reason to stay with Adam when he tries to subjugate her, and is indifferent to the threats of force, even by angels. The narration becomes like a jilted lover's story when her new lover is said to be a demon, and her story trails off rather than following the fate of her many children.

God is apparently not happy with Eve or Lilith and curses all of humanity because of Eve's sin of persuading Adam to taste the fruit of knowledge. According to the Bible story, God tries creating women a couple of times and decides they are unruly seductresses ruining His plans. Maybe the problem wasn't them? Maybe the problem was in the recounting and later patriarchal attempt to minimize the power of the maternal in all her manifestations.

Mothering has no beginning or end. Mothering is a constant flow of giving and receiving love. It is a state of being and an energy always in some phase of creation, reflecting a continuous cycle of being born and dying. Within all our mothering experiences there are phases and junctures where we come together and acknowledge what is so in that moment. When we get too fixated on a linear progression of events through a life cycle, it creates scarcity of time, and it has no reality or meaning other than what we give it.

There is a Lilith hiding in every manifestation of the Mother Code, an echo from our past as revered creators placed at the center of our societies. The system that has replaced the last matricentric age has shown us endless war, environmental degradation, slavery, and a general disregard for life and human dignity. Maybe we would have been better off had Adam just let Lilith be his equal. What we have from Adam and Eve is a planet on fire and in a state of perpetual war.

Find your inner Lilith. Find the women at the margins of your story, people who have been erased but have left a small trace behind. It might be a great-aunt who never married and was whispered about by the family. It could be a cousin you never see at family gatherings. Or a friend from your circle of friends who sort of disappeared, and nobody knows what happened to her. Or she could be in a book or a film or a chapter of history. Amazing, radical, powerful women have been a problem for our society for a long time. Find them. They have something very important to say about the way we live—and the way we should live.

REFLECTION

Connect with your Lilith voice. Have a dialogue with her.

Ask her what is out of balance in your life.

Discuss what needs to be spoken that will bring you into alignment with your Mother Code.

Your inner Lilith knows what you most need, and I urge you to take one step toward it.

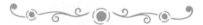

Whether you look through the lens of Arthurian legend, the Bible, or your own experience of motherhood. Whether you are in the midst of mothering a toddler, a teenager, or a career. Whether you have always considered yourself a vessel of expansive energy, or whether this is the first time you are hearing the possibility. Wherever you are at this moment, it is perfect, and I invite you into all the possibilities that mothering can bring to you. I beckon you to open yourself to the deep primal calling that invites you to take on the sacred mantel of mothering as a gift to yourself and a gift to those closest to you and beyond.

The 2022 Nobel Prize for physics revealed the mind-blowing reality that the universe is not locally real and how data is shared across distances in ways that counteract everything we previously thought. I am not a physicist, but I wonder what applying this paradigm-shifting reality to conscious mothering would bring to our world. When ancient wisdom is proven by science, we get people's attention. From 1940 to 1990, studies of quantum foundations were considered "philosophy" and even "crackpottery." Our human wiring initially perceives expansive awareness as threatening, so we do everything from minimizing to criticizing to hide it, like standing in an earthquake with buildings toppling down around us and pretending it is just another normal day.

Eventually, we come around, but we are at a time in history where putting our heads in the sand when we know how to do things differently has dire consequences. Even knowing and experiencing the unleashing of mother energy into the world would ultimately bring peace, connection, and abundance to our world, we resist because a sick system is a familiar system. Until enough of us brave souls use our voices to bring a new reality into being, we will experience more and more dire consequences. I stand with you as you make this choice and join the mothering revolution.

As we honor the real mothering of ourselves, we can reflect and radiate to others, giving them permission to honor and live expansively in the sacredness of all the aspects of mothering—allowing, tending, and being. Matriarchal means good for all. If we embraced caring for all, imagine the love that would build and build exponentially.

We have discussed many varieties of mothering across time. Another practice I want to mention from these bygone eras was for women to have a child, but then have them fostered in another household. There were many reasons for this practice that ranged from being sent away for specific training, to keeping their identity secret for protective reasons, to the true parentage of the child, one that would bring shame to the family. At first, I was appalled and judged this behavior as unmotherly and irresponsible.

But then I remembered that we are merely a portal for our children to enter this world and stewards to help them become who they are meant to be. They are not our property. As you practice living your Mother Code and continue to build and deepen a sense of self along with your children, you are also preparing *yourself* for them leaving. There are many "leavings" through the moments of motherhood—they leave your body, they leave your breast, they go to day-care, then school, they build friendships outside the home, they need you less and less, and then one day they leave your home for good. Orienting to the Cosmic Codes guides you in creating and building a sense of self that prepares you to release your children into the world and, at the same time, be excited for this next phase of your life. Loving them like mad as you simultaneously let them go is the story of a mother.

Rite of Passage—Third Trimester

Let these stories of and possibilities for the manifestation of mother energy vibrate within you. Can you feel the energy? What sensations do you feel in your body? You may not have words for what you are experiencing, but let it resonate. With the pain, there is joy. Amid tragedy, there is love. Love, love, and more love. That pours out of a mother. A mother is a vessel of love.

What is mother energy?

Mother energy is fierce
Mother energy is creation
Mother energy is determination
Mother energy is deep
Mother energy is vast
Mother energy is pain
Mother energy never gives up
Mother energy is LOVE
Mother energy is YOU!
YOU are LOVE!

You are all of this and more! You have infinite choices on how you express, share, and embody your mother energy. You have endless amounts of it, there is no end to the creative expression of you.

Conclusion

"What's your intention for the Temazcal?" I asked Lara as we drove to Lupita's jungle home outside of Zihuatanejo in Mexico.

With a mix of peaceful and nervous anticipation, Lara responded, "Oh wow, hmm...I feel pretty raw, open, and blessed from our day together." After a thoughtful pause, she said with a big grin and almost devious laugh, "I am thinking...let's go to the cosmos! Why not, right? Why not open myself to even more wisdom and healing and surrender—with the Universe. I intend to surrender to the medicine of the Temazcal!"

Now that is an intention! And it felt right on point for Lara based on the progression of our day together. Having immersed herself in deeply personal activations I had curated for her to regenerate, reawaken, and realign with the wisdom and mysteries of the womb, it felt like an oddly normal next step for our day together.

After holding space for Lara while also on my internal journey as facilitator, I similarly felt it was time to hop into the rocket ship of transcendent experience that only the contained space of intense heat, steam, chanting, and drumming of a Temazcal could evoke. Our day together had opened spaces for Lara that beheld rewriting her own birth story, visualizing and communicating with the children her womb would hold one day, as well as healing that unlocked a soft sensual power within her womb. So had we not done another thing that day, her experience would have felt complete.

Lupita, a well-known local healer and medicine woman, welcomed us into her space with her big smile and open arms. She guided us to where she had set up for the opening ritual. With the sacred smoke of copal pouring over us, we readied ourselves by cleansing and releasing any negative energy that may have hindered our experience. As Lupita blew through the conch shell, we raised our hands in gratitude and praise to the spirits of the four directions. We moved to our hands and knees and put our foreheads directly on Mother Earth, honoring the five elements—earth, air, fire, water, and space.

I love this ritual and deeply honor the value of acknowledging Source, so why was I finding it unusually difficult to keep myself present? I caught myself going through the motions and realized so much was swirling in my mind from the spaces we evoked through the day. How could I open myself to more when I already felt so full? (I later found out Lara was feeling the same way.)

"Trust the process and stay open," I told myself.

I focused in and listened more with my heart and less with my head as Lupita described the Temazcal as the Sacred Womb and portal that both brings forth life through birth and releases life through death. A pre-Hispanic practice that had been forbidden for centuries during colonization is once again providing healing medicine for anyone who goes inside.

Having made this choice many times over the past ten years of coming to this region, this was not my first time hearing this from her. But somehow, it was feeling different. I was shifting from *understanding* the Temazcal as a metaphoric womb and expanding into intuitive *knowing* that showed me the real nature of the space of creation.

Lupita invited us to ask permission of the ancestors before we crawled into the already warm and dark space. We found our places inside; it always amazes me how what looks like such a small space from the outside is so spacious and expansive inside. Being that we were all women, she invited us to remove our bathing suits, as was the ancient practice. While still a little uncomfortable for me, I knew the freedom that comes from removing all unnecessary barriers. So off went my bathing suit!

After stating our intentions—both having our own version that included letting go of control, opening ourselves to wisdom, and flying to the cosmos, she put water with healing herbs in it onto the hot stones. Steam filled the space. I felt the heat envelop me. Lupita chanted in Spanish. It was beginning.

After the first chant, it was time to close the opening at the top of the domed structure to create total darkness. Lupita asked one of us to do it since we are tall. Lara, a 6-foot Division 1 volleyball champion, jumped up to do the honors. Then, as she was about to put the pillow in the hole, she let out a loud scream.

"AHHH! OHHH! I stepped on glass! Or coals? Something is burning me! Oh my god, the pain!" she exclaimed.

At first glance, the floor was completely clear. No glass, no fire. What happened?

Lara continued to cry out in pain when Sara, Lupita's assistant, spotted a scorpion scurrying across the floor. I saw it also, and in a quick moment, Sara threw a towel on it and stepped on it to end its life. Lupita was visibly aghast, saying that in 14 years, she had never seen a scorpion in her Temazcal. She also made sure to tell us later she blessed the scorpion and thanked it for its life.

"So much for going to the cosmos," I thought. Our intention was taken by this tiny pest! Or was it?

Lara went right to her logical brain.

"What's going to happen to me? What do we do? I usually swell up when I am bitten or stung. Do we go to the hospital?" she asked. Being an elite athlete, Lara was no stranger to pain, so I was not surprised when she went to concrete problem solving as her initial way of dealing with this painful circumstance.

Lupita and Sara shared the information regarding scorpion stings. They would monitor her breathing and look for unusual swelling. If nothing changed and her throat didn't start closing, she would not need to go to the hospital.

"It hurts so much!! My foot feels like it is on fire. I have never felt anything this painful, but yes, I can breathe fine, and nothing is changing in my throat," she responded when asked during the important minutes post-sting.

When it became clear Lara was not having an allergic reaction, Lupita asked permission to work with her. Without hesitation, Lara replied, "Yes!" She chose to surrender to the journey. She said yes to the mystery and unknown of what was to come.

Our Stories

The role of storytelling in ancient societies cannot be overstated. Without a written record, the survival of cultural identity, beliefs, and practices depended on the ability of storytellers to capture and convey the essence of their community's experiences. These stories were often told in communal settings, creating a shared experience that reinforced social bonds and a collective memory. Myths, legends, and folktales served as tools for explaining the world, from the origins of the universe to the reason behind natural phenomena. Storytelling was a dynamic, living tradition, adaptable to the needs and circumstances of the community, ensuring its relevance across time.

On one level, Lara's story revealed once again that our brains are wired to keep us alive. This is evolution. It is wonderful and it is limiting. The truth is we have had many, many, many, more years of a brain dedicated to solving the problem of keeping us alive and relatively few years exploring the problem of how to *thrive* in the life we live in a meaningful and fulfilling way.

Lara didn't know what would happen when she said yes to Lupita's invitation, but she sensed, tapped into her intuition, and trusted—herself and the community that surrounded her. By staying in the present moment, Lara is rewiring her default circuitry and living a new story. This story will find its place among other women doing the same, and this collective of rewritten stories will bring into balance his-story with her-story.

For thousands of years, men's stories have dominated the public sphere. They have been the ones to tell the grand narratives— the tales of heroes, wars, and the exploits of gods and kings. These stories were celebrated and passed down in formal settings, often to reinforce the values of a patriarchal society. They focused on external achievements, conquest, and resolution of conflict—things seen as the domain of men. This isn't just a reflection of men's experiences but also a way of framing what is considered important, valuable, and worth remembering.

Women have often been the keepers of the private, domestic stories—those centered on relationships, community, and the rhythms of daily life. These stories, rich with emotional depth and moral lessons, were shared in intimate settings, often within the home or in women-only spaces. They reflected women's insight into the emotional and social fabric of the human experience. But because these stories were not told in the public sphere, they were often dismissed as less significant and less worthy of preservation.

This marginalization of women's voices in storytelling has had profound consequences. It has shaped our collective memory in ways that focus on men's experiences and achievements while relegating women's stories to the background. As I shared earlier, written language further entrenched this disparity. As stories moved from the fluid, adaptable oral tradition to the fixed form of the written word, those in power—often men—decided which stories were worth recording. This led to the canonization of certain narratives, while others were lost or forgotten.

The shift from oral and pictorial storytelling to written language also marked a shift in control. People who could read and write—typically a privileged, educated few—gained the power to define culture and history. Women, who were often denied access to education, found their stories pushed further into the margins. The written word allowed for the preservation of complex ideas and narratives, but it also meant that women's voices, which had thrived in the oral tradition, were further silenced.

Yet, the importance of women's stories cannot be overstated. They offer perspectives on life, love, community, and resilience that are essential to a full understanding of the human experience. They challenge the notion that only grand, public events are worthy of remembrance. Today, as we continue to fight for gender equality, reclaiming these stories is important. It's about recognizing that the personal is political and that the everyday experiences of women are as valuable and important as the exploits of men. This isn't just about adding women's stories to the narrative; it's about rethinking what we consider important, who gets to tell the story, and how we make sure everyone's voice is heard.

When my mother first shared with me her stories of the series of traumas she endured through her twenties, she was embarrassed and immediately had regret. She assumed I would think badly of her because that is what a culture that casts a shadow of shame on our lived experiences would have us do. I felt nothing resembling shame—only compassion and profound sadness she had kept all of this inside rather than brought it out into the open where it could be healed. I said it then and feel it even more now that her revealing of this raw, deeply vulnerable, and painful aspect of her life's journey was a priceless gift.

For it was in sharing her story that I came to know myself. And it is in passing our stories to our daughters and sons so they too can know themselves. Extending beyond our families, the story of women's pain, in all its manifestations, is the ongoing story of all life on this planet.

The marginalized stories of women's lived experience, either erased or altered to suit the prevailing culture, are emerging from the shadows and hidden places. For now, we can be satisfied that the start of such a movement seems to be reaching a wider audience through historical fiction.

It took a book by Dan Brown, *The Da Vinci Code*, and subsequent movie starring Tom Hanks to remind the world of the complex identity of Mary Magdalene. This figure appears in the New Testament with the kind of ambiguity from questionable and incomplete elision that led us to Lilith in the Old Testament. If one reads the totality of texts produced about Jesus in the first couple hundred years after his death, there is a preponderance of evidence that Mary Magdalene played a large role in Jesus' ministry and that she was his wife.[1]

Further, some accounts refer to their children.

Women have not fared well in the religion founded in the name of Jesus Christ (emphasis on "in the name of" as no evidence points to his desire to found a new religion—that was incorrectly written into the story). And while much of this intolerance comes from the beginning, the excision of Mary Magdalene, along with many other aspects of the life of Jesus and his more esoteric teachings, began with the aggressive censorship of the texts written about both. The Bible is important because of the stories it tells and its teachings. It is also notable for what it leaves out.

Mary Magdalene presented as the wife of Jesus must have

---

1 *Smithsonian Magazine* published an extensive account of the complex history of Mary Magdalene here: https://www.smithsonianmag.com/history/who-was-mary-magdalene-119565482/.

enraged the early Christian misogynists. Imagine a story of Jesus in which he is in full partnership with a woman, having children with her, choosing her as a leader, and entrusting his legacy to her. It makes perfect sense, yet she has been relegated to a minor role and a misrepresented one in the Bible as it appears today. That was a deliberate decision, and we can even say where and when the decision to cut her out was made.

Mary represents the human side of Jesus. Even in the accepted texts of the New Testament, Mary is the person who washes Jesus' body after crucifixion, clear evidence she was married to him, as the body of a rabbi, which he was considered, would not have been touched by anyone else (except perhaps someone closely related to him). Her presence in this capacity provides powerful evidence of the spiritual significance of women which even centuries of patriarchal editing could not altogether erase. If, as the Gospel of Mary suggests, she was most beloved of his followers, and if this provoked jealousy and in-fighting by his other disciples, this scene would be familiar to many women.

Further, would it be so far-fetched to imagine that a religious teacher who emphasizes the needy and the poor would turn to a woman to spread that message, especially if she proved to be intelligent and capable of leading?

It was divine timing. I read the *Madonna Secret,* by Sophie Strand, when I started on the journey of writing this book. It was the most resonate retelling of the story of Mary Magdalene and Jesus I have come across. I feel it speaks to all of our mother lines and how much we need to intuit our way through the history that has been rewritten to serve a dominant culture.

There is much more that can be said about this topic, but the key point I want to convey is that the marginalization of Mary Magdalene is one more instance of a woman with a powerful story in history being pushed to the margins. The gospel associated with her is a compelling read in part because it introduces some interesting theological ideas that resonate with the concepts in this book, but that's a story for another time.

The Magic of the Mother Code

When we think about the Mother Code and the path by which it came to be what it is today, it is worthwhile to consider how hard mostly men have had to work to create and defend a worldview that pushes women, and especially mothers, to the fringes. Yet mothers, like water, always find a way. We know Mary just as we know so many before and after her. I believe that there has always been a glitch in the Mother Code that points the way back to the communion of all of us in a much more peaceful and prosperous world, one that honors our contributions and celebrates the powerful women who have come before us.

There will be throughlines that carry into all phases of motherhood; unique joys and challenges will come into focus at various inflection points in your and your children's developmental milestones. I implore you to stay as focused on orienting to the present with yourself and your child(ren) as possible. Still, it is helpful to see glimpses and foreshadowing of what it looks like to apply this methodology to upcoming stages of motherhood. I hope to pique your interest and understanding that the muscles you are building now will continue to get stronger and open the door to so much richness and so many possibilities for YOU in these years you are dedicating to birthing your dreams and mothering another human.

If we go back to Lara's experience, our first response collectively was to solve the problem of a dangerous and potentially life-threatening situation. Unless you live in an area where scorpions are common, most of us would assume that a scorpion sting meant a trip to the hospital. Once she had the data she needed to make an informed choice, the question became *how* she would interact with the no longer life-threatening pain.

I was so glad it was Lara, a woman who has traversed the land-scape of healing and self-actualization with the same dedication she had given her volleyball career earlier in life. I expected she would not only be up for an expanded experience but also had the training to navigate it. And to be clear, had Lara shown even an inkling of an allergic reaction or strong desire to go to the hospital, we would not have hesitated to transfer her.

I thought about some other women I know who would have had a very different reaction. Their fear would have shut down any possibility of entertaining the concept that other options existed for this experience. It would have looked more like Lara saying, "I blow up with stings! Take me to the hospital immediately!" This is a perfectly valid choice in a moment where pain and fear collide. What I want you to consider is that more than one choice exists. There are additional valid responses that may not seem im-mediately viable and come more from an intuitive, body-centered place. These choices have the potential to provide healing beyond the physical to include the emotional, spiritual, and psychological.

What followed after Lara saying yes to Lupita's invitation to an alternative experience in lieu of a perfunctory shot at a hospital was a spontaneous shamanic healing. Lupita was having a tobacco cere-mony that night, so she had sacred healing tobacco at the ready. (This coincidence was not lost on us!) I had always held Lupita as a wise woman and healer, but I had never seen her like this.

This was a woman channeling the wisdom of ancient healing. Smoke from the sacred tobacco was blown onto and into Lara. Alternately, Lara was asked to take the tobacco in herself but not inhale it because of the dizzying effects. They both spit a lot which happens in this releasing experience and signifies letting go of negative energy. Lupita poured rubbing alcohol on her; she put it on cotton balls and placed them in Lara's ears. The sounds and words they shared were unidentifiable but familiar from times I had entered altered states.

Time stood still, and we were lifted out of consensual reality into a profound journey of cosmic proportions.

I stood as witness, holding space, and physically held Lara at various points. Lupita and I made eye contact several times, and without words, she guided me on how best to help. It was so clear that Lupita was the midwife with Sara and I as a doula guiding Lara through a shamanic initiation and rebirth.

I was observing Lupita as she opened herself to be guided by her intuition and partner with Spirit—something I have been aspiring to do in my own healing practice. She was not following a one-size-fits-all checklist of transactional procedures—she was lockstepping through so she could move on to the next person in the waiting room. She was 100% there for Lara and held a solid, grounded space that created massive trust and security, just as my midwife held me in her gaze when I was terrified to push into the pain. I knew she had me covered, and the embrace of her presence gave me the security to bypass my hijacked brain.

These are the conditions that create a launching pad for your spirit to soar and discover new aspects of yourself.

When you rewrite your Mother Codes and own the Cosmic Codes, you no longer live the same story repeatedly. You surrender and merge with the ongoing creation of all that is. You become a part of herstory—the enduring story of the power of love—living love, sharing love, joining in love, birthing with love, mothering everyone and everything with love.

Is it a coincidence that a full rainbow spread her glorious arch behind me as I was writing this conclusion? Heavens no! At this point, we are well beyond even considering such basic misinterpretations! I immediately ran outside to open myself to what this portent held for me.

Was it a transmission, an invitation or an affirmation? Yes! It was all of it.

This mystical gift can be explained by science, but we no longer reduce it to such basic terms. Now, instead, we have the choice to remember the cosmic code we are one with the universe. Crowned by this rainbow of my becoming, I am invited to live the dreams this rainbow holds—the realities that I have yet to grasp but I am on the path to discover continuously, for there is no end to this journey.

When you acknowledge the illusion and the life-shrinking danger of the Mother Codes, you are free. Free to create the motherhood of your choosing. Freedom is as exhilarating as it is terrifying. Our safe and known reality of motherhood is the prism. Our cosmic motherhood is available when we shine the light of truth on our prism and reveal the colors that open us to beautiful perspectives that were always right there inside. We forgot how to access them. We "know" what happens when the light hits it, but are only beginning to KNOW it, to own it as our reflection.

Once you welcome this light and experience glimpses of this new reality, I share a word of caution. When you stretch beyond what you ever thought possible, you may protect your gains. This is a place where you risk settling into this new normal. Yes, you have manifested the vision you once thought was out of reach. By all means, do celebrate. Revel and enjoy it for a time. And then I invite you to consider staying on the journey of the continued birthing of yourself.

When the healing experience brought on by the sting of a scorpion felt complete, Lupita broke out into a huge smile. She looked at Lara and me and asked, "Are you ready?"

She saw the questioning looks on our faces and said, "Yes, are you ready for the Temazcal now?"

Our jaws dropped. Talking on top of each other, we both were like, "What?? Really? Are you joking? Wasn't that incredible initiatic rebirth our experience for the evening? We feel more than served!"

She was not joking. She was serious. She assured us that the space had been inspected and we could carry on with the Temazcal. OK, but wasn't she exhausted? How did she even have the energy to continue pouring herself into us? This was an invitation to the next level of trust and surrender.

Before we could overthink it and let fear of further scorpion encounters or guilt that we were taking up too much of her time and energy stop us, we both said yes and re-entered the Temazcal. The steaming heat and medicinal herbs felt like a warm blanket wrapping itself around us. The rhythmic drumbeat and beautiful voices of Lupita and Sara opened a space for us to integrate what we had been through. Lara and I agreed afterward that we felt cradled in the arms of a loving mother. Our gratitude for the entire experience was immeasurable.

Motherhood, similarly, isn't comprised of one dramatic initiation that makes you a mother. Conception, pregnancy, and birth are merely the warm-ups foreshadowing a lifetime of initiatic re-birth experiences that open you to becoming a mother. As existential philosopher Simone de Beauvoir says, "One is not born, but rather, becomes a woman."

To embrace one's new vision of oneself as a mother and let the old cues fade away, and to do so using the energy of your fear to propel you forward: This is the mental state that best describes the active, maturing, unceasing process of Rewriting the Mother Code. You are ready. You have always been ready.

Blessings on your journey.

Acknowledgements

I have come to discover that all books are love stories. Love is the seed and the nourishment that fosters an idea to take shape. Through myriad love affairs, my thoughts and ideas have taken form, and they are offered with love to you, the reader.

I am wildly grateful for the steadfast, solid, and ever present current of human love given to me by my husband Rich. Our wedding vows set an intention for us to grow as partners, lovers, and best friends, and it is only through the ups and downs of living into that vision that this story has unfolded. You are a magnificent man, and I am beyond grateful for all the ways you express your love for me.

For my daughters, Morgan and Hannah, I am forever grateful that you answered our invitation and chose us as your parents, and my womb for your doorway into this world. Thank you for both for being exquisitely yourselves and igniting my life with so much love and wisdom.

I would not be here to have this human experience were it not for the union of my mother, Dorothy, and my father, Frank.

Your dance of relationship brought me into being and formed me through my childhood. Thank you for being the perfect parents for my soul's development. I have extra-special gratitude to my mother for bestowing the gift of her vulnerable story to me and giving me permission to share it.

Writing a book is raw and intimate and you need people you feel safe with to bring your story and passion out into the world. Much like midwives, my publisher, Kristen McGuiness, editor, Jamie Lou; book coach, Jennifer Loudan; and editor/consultant Gabriel Piemonte shared their literary expertise and infused me with the confidence that I had everything I needed inside of me to birth this book. Thank you for believing in me and guiding me—in your own unique and profound ways—through many moments of fear and doubt. I cannot imagine having done this without you all. Extra shout out to Gabriel for being a real-life guardian angel by my side starting with my dissertation, then chapters in Demeter Press, and now this book.

True sisterhood is priceless. I have a blessing of riches when it comes to women in my life who are solid allies and chosen sisters. You have been my shining lights through thick and thin. To Barbara for pouring encouragement, positive vibes, and love into me when I need it most (which is basically daily!) Thank you for your genuine care and inspiration as a feminine force in the world. To my forever sister Jennifer—my guardian angel in this life and beyond. Thank you for guiding me on my path as my chosen big sister. Your spirit is infused in these pages. To Denise and Edda: We have been through so much together, and I wouldn't be the woman I am without you both.

To Mary Sommers for midwifing both of my daughters into the world and empowering me to access my innate wisdom through the process. You are a rare gem, and I am grateful for the loving space you continue to hold for me and my becoming.

To the Ladies of the Pond (Barbara, Michele, Alison, Deb, Ela) who ventured to Woodstock with me when I gave birth to the full

first draft of my book. To the newly forming Goddess Council—
Aine and Sophia for opening doors and possibilities that will continue to emerge and grow.

To each of my podcast guests and clients for trusting me as well
as being a catalyst of my own continued transformation. To the
women who have joined me in my retreats, taken workshops with
me, invited me into their birthing journeys, you amazing women
who believe in me and have been moved by my mission and my
vision, you are in every chapter, in every word. I send you all my
loving gratitude. Extra shout out to the women who participated
in my doctoral curriculum evaluation study. Your participation
gave quantitative and qualitative evidence and reflected the desire
and need for this message to get out into the world.

To the formidable community of women in academia: Women
working together is the most powerful force humanity has seen!
Thank you all so much. You have made me better, and you have cer-
tainly improved my work. Special thanks to Dr. Andrea O'Reilly,
founder of Demeter Press, and Katie Garner, Director of IAMAS
(International Association of Maternal Action and Scholarship),
who have been an integral part of honing so many of my ideas.

I am grateful for the support and teamwork of so many loving
hands that make Rewrite the Mother Code, LLC, an ongoing reality. Thank you to Jessica Zweig and the team at SimplyBe agency
for launching me into the world. To Alexia Vernon for gently
nudging out my first keynote talk and providing ongoing business
support. To Jonathan Stancato for illuminating a path for my voice
to be heard in the world. To Ashley Weller-Donahue for stepping
in and wrapping your arms around all the pieces of the business
to make them a unified whole. To Fearless Foundry for taking
me and my brand to the next level of depth and sophistication.
To the team at Rise Books for applying your heads and hearts to
make this book a reality. I couldn't wish for a more effective, more
supportive team to help me get to this point.

To James Kawainui, Stacy Levy, Julie Ryan, Nada Yousif, David Elliot, Michael Nourse, and Sophia Trevanna for sharing your gifts of intuitive wisdom and guidance to keep me aligned with my mission and purpose. For all my past therapists, coaches, and practitioners, I thank you for the integral part you played in my journey and development.

I am grateful for the land that held me, spoke to me, and mothered me throughout the year of writing this book. I have intended along the way that the energy of these magical places is infused in the book and will be felt by anyone who reads it. I will use their current names, but I also wish to thank and honor the original peoples of each of these places: Chicago, IL; Zihuatanejo, Mexico; Ojai, CA; Woodstock, NY; Malta; Dooks, Ireland; Paris, France; and numerous places in Iceland.

The Cosmic Codes were my lived experience as I set about this quest. I am grateful for my ever-expanding relationship with the Divine Mother and humbled at the opportunity to be a conduit of Your wisdom. Even when I was physically alone. You were by my side every moment.

I have been blessed by nurturing, comfort, support, loving, and occasionally the much needed kicks in the butt from so many people it would take another book to hold them all. Even what I have expressed falls short of the gushing appreciation I am filled with. It is my wish that if you are not specifically named you know you are part of this love story, and I am bursting with gratitude for the big and small ways you have touched me on my journey.

Bibliography

Apple, Rima. *Perfect Motherhood: Science and Childrearing in America.* Rutgers University Press, 2006.

Arendell, Terry. "Conceiving and Investigating Motherhood: The Decade's Scholarship." *Journal of Marriage and Family* 62: 1192-1207.

Arendell, Terry. "Conceiving and Investigating Motherhood: The Decade's Scholarship." *Journal of Marriage and Family* 62, no. 4 (2000): 1192-1207.

Barlow, Constance A., and Kathleen V. Cairns. "Mothering as a Psychological Experience: A Grounded Theory Exploration." *Canadian Journal of Counselling* 31, no. 3 (1997): 232-247.

Beauvoir, Simone de. "The Second Sex." *Classic and Contemporary Readings in Sociology.* Routledge, 2014. 118-123.

Benes, Francine M., Jill Bolte Taylor, and Miles C. Cunningham. "Convergence and Plasticity of Monoaminergic Systems in the Medial Prefrontal Cortex during the Postnatal Period: Implications for the Development of Psychopathology." *Cerebral Cortex* 10, no. 10 (2000): 1014-1027.

Block, Joyce. *Motherhood as Metamorphosis: Change and Continuity in the Life of a New Mother.* Dutton, 1990.

Boucai, Liat, and Rachel Karniol. "Suppressing and Priming the Motivation for Motherhood." *Sex Roles* (Springer), 2008: 851-870.

Bowlby, John. *A Secure Base: Parent-Child Attachment and Healthy Human Development.* Basic Books, 1988.

Cabo, Mariana Costa do, et al., eds. "Fifty Years After 'Good Enough' Donald Woods Winnicott (1896-1971)." *Jornal Brasileiro de Psiquiatria* 71, no. 1 (2022): 3-4.

Cambridge Editors. *Cambridge Content Dictionary.* Cambridge University Press, 2008.

Caplan, Paula, and Ian Hall-McCorquodale. "Mother-blaming in Major Clinical Journals." *American Journal of Orthopsychiatry*, 1985: 345-353.

Chodorow, Nancy. "The Psychodynamics of the Family." *The Second Wave: A Reader in Feminist Theory*, edited by Linda Nicholson, Psychology Press, 1997, pp. 181-197.

Chown, Marcus. *The Magic Furnace: The Search for the Origins of Atoms.* Random House, 2011.

Cummins, Molly Wiant. "Miracles and Home Births: The Importance of Media Representations of Birth." *Critical Studies in Media Communication* 37, no. 1 (2020): 85-96.

Daines, Chantel L., et al. "Effects of Positive and Negative Childhood Experiences on Adult Family Health." *BMC Public Health* 21 (2021): 1-8.

Damasio, Antonio R. *The Feeling of What Happens: Body, Emotion, and the Making of Consciousness.* Harcourt Brace, 1999.

Douglas, Susan and Meredith Michaels. *The Mommy Myth: The Idealization of Motherhood and How it Has Undermined All Women.* Free Press, 2004.

Downe, Susan, ed. *Normal Childbirth: Evidence and Debate.* Elsevier Health Sciences, 2008.

Duarte-Guterman, Paula, Benedetta Leuner, and Liisa AM Galea. "The Long and Short Term Effects of Motherhood on the Brain." *Frontiers in Neuroendocrinology* 53 (2019): 100740.

Dudenhausen, Joachim W., Amos Grunebaum, and Ursula M. Staudinger. "Optimization of Women's Health Before Conception When Pregnancy Has Been Postponed." *Journal of Perinatal Medicine* 41, no. 1 (2013).

Dwek, Carol. *Mindset: The New Psychology of Success.* Ballantine Books, 2007.

Eberhard-Gran, Malin, et al. "Postnatal Care: A Cross-cultural and Historical Perspective." *Archives of Women's Mental Health* 13 (2010): 459-466.

Ennis, Linda Rose. *Intensive Mothering: The Cultural Contradictions of Modern Motherhood*. Demeter Press, 2014.

Faulkner, Sandra. "Bad Mom(my) Litany: Spanking Cultural Myths of Middle-Class Motherhood." Cultural Studies-Critical Methodologies (Sage), 2014: 138-146.

Flexner, Abraham. "Medical Education in the United States and Canada." *Bulletin of the World Health Organization* 80 (2002): 594-602.

Fosha, Diana. "Emotion and Recognition at Work: Energy, Vitality, Pleasure, Truth, Desire & The Emergent Phenomenology of Transformational Experience." *The Healing Power of Emotions*. Norton, 2009.

Galinsky, Ellen. *The Six Stages of Parenthood*. New York: Merlyond Lawrence, 1987.

Gaskin, Ina May. *Spiritual Midwifery*. Book Publishing Company, 2010.

Gilligan, Carol. *In a Different Voice: Psychological Theory and Women's Development*. Harvard University Press, 1993.

Gopnik, Alison. *The Gardener and the Carpenter*. Farrar, Straus and Giroux, 2016.

Harding, M. Esther. *The Way of All Women*. Shambhala, 1990.

Hays, Sharon. *The Cultural Contradictions of Motherhood*. Yale University Press, 1996.

Heffner, Elaine. *Mothering: The Emotional Experience of Motherhood After Freud and Feminism*. Doubleday Anchor, 1980.

Hrdy, Sarah Blaffer. *Mothers and Others: The Evolutionary Origins of Mutual Understanding*. Harvard University Press, 2009.

Iacoboni, Marco. "Imitation, Empathy, and Mirror Neurons." *Annual Review of Psychology* 60 (2009): 653-70.

Johnston, Deirdre, and Debra Swanson. "Constructing the 'Good Mother': The Experience of Mothering Ideologies by Work Status." *Sex Roles* 54, no. 7 (2006): 509-519.

Karr-Morse, Robin, and Meridith Wiley. *Ghosts from the Nursery: Tracing the Roots of Violence*. Atlantic Monthly Press, 2014.

Kawash, Samira. "New Directions in Motherhood Studies." *Signs: Journal of Women in Culture and Society* 36, no. 4 (2011): 969-1003.

Lankford, Valerie. "The Parent Ego State from a Reparenting Perspective." *Transactional Analysis Journal* 18 (1988): 47-50.

Leap, Nicky, and Tricia Anderson. "The Role of Pain in Normal Birth and the Empowerment of Women." *Normal Childbirth: Evidence and Debate* 29 (2008).

Leifer, Myra. "Psychological Effects of Motherhood: A Study of First Pregnancy." New York, Praeger Publishers, 1980.

Liss, Miriam, Holly Schiffrin, and Kathryn Rizzo. "Maternal Guilt and Shame: The Role of Self-discrepancy and Fear of Negative Evaluation." *Journal of Child and Family Studies* 22, no. 8 (2013): 1112-1119.

Liss, Miriam, Holly Schiffrin, Virginia Mackintosh, Haley Miles-McLean, and Mindy Erchull. "Development and Validation of a Quantitative Measure of Intensive Parenting Attitudes." *Journal of Child and Family Studies* 22, no. 5 (2013): 621-636.

Louden, Jennifer. *Pregnant Woman's Comfort Book: A Self-Nurturing Guide to Your Emotional Well-Being During Pregnancy and Early Motherhood.* Harper Collins, 2005.

Lundsberg, Lisbet S., et al. "Knowledge, Attitudes, and Practices regarding Conception and Fertility: A Population-based Survey among Reproductive-age United States Women." *Fertility and Sterility* 101, no. 3 (2014): 767-774.

Lyons, Gertrude. *Expanding Mothering: Raising a Woman's Awareness of the Opportunities for Personal and Psychosocial Growth and Development in Mothering—A Curriculum Evaluation Study.* 2017. Wright Graduate University, Ed.D. dissertation.

Martin, Lee, and Bo Shao. "Early Immersive Culture Mixing: The Key to Understanding Cognitive and Identity Differences among Multiculturals." *Journal of Cross-Cultural Psychology* 47, no. 10 (2016): 1409-1429.

Maushart, Susan. *The Mask of Motherhood: How Becoming a Mother Changes Our Lives and Why We Never Talk About It.* Penguin Books, 2000.

McBride, Angela Barron. *The Growth and Development of Mothers.* Harper and Row, 1973.

McVeigh, Carol. "Motherhood Experiences from the Perspective of First Time Mothers." *Clinical Nursing Research* 6, no. 4 (Nov 1997): 335-348.

Mercer, Ramona T., Glen C. Doyle, and Elizabeth G. Nichols. *Transitions In A Woman's Life. Vol. 12.* Springer Publishing Co., 1989.

Miller, Tina. "'Is This What Motherhood Is All About?' Weaving Experiences and Discourse through Transition to First-Time Motherhood." *Gender & Society* 21, no. 3 (2007): 337-358.

Murkoff, Heidi. *What to Expect When You're Expecting.* Workman Publishing, 2016.

Noble, Vicki. *Motherpeace: A Way to the Goddess through Myth, Art and Tarot.* Harper & Row, 1983.

Odent, Michel. "The Masculinisation of the Birth Environment." *Journal of Prenatal & Perinatal Psychology & Health* 23, no. 3 (2009).

Olsen, Mark, and Samuel Avital. *The Conception Mandala: Creative Techniques for Inviting a Child Into Your Life.* Inner Traditions/Bear & Co., 1992.

O'Reilly, Andrea, ed. *Mother Matters: Motherhood as Discourse and Practice: Essays from the Journal of the Association for Research on Mothering.* Association for Research on Mothering, 2004.

O'Reilly, Andrea, ed. *Mother Outlaws: Theories and Practices of Empowered Mothering.* Canadian Scholars Press, 2004.

O'Reilly, Andrea, ed. *Twenty-first Century Motherhood: Experience, Identity, Policy, Agency*. Columbia University Press, 2010.

Palkovitz, Rob, Loren Marks, David Appleby, and Erin Holmes. "Parenting and Adult Development: Contexts, Processes and Products of Intergenerational Relationships." *Faculty Publications and Presentations*. Paper 9, July 2002.

Pert, Candace. *Molecules Of Emotion: The Science Behind Mind-Body Medicine*. Simon & Schuster, 1999.

Prinds, Christina, Niels Christian Hvidt, Ole Mogensen, and Niels Buus. "Making Existential Meaning in Transition to Motherhood—A Scoping Review." *Midwifery* 30, no. 6 (2014): 733-741.

Rich, Adrienne. *Of Woman Born: Motherhood as Experience and Institution*. W.W. Norton, 1995.

Ricks, Shirley. "Father-Infant Interactions: A Review of Empirical Research." *Family Relations*, no. 34 (1985): 505-511.

Rizzato, Matteo and Davide Donelli. *I Am Your Mirror: Mirror Neurons and Empathy*. Torino: Blossoming Books, 2014.

Rizzo, Kathryn, Holly Schiffrin, and Miriam Liss. "Insight into the Parenthood Paradox: Mental Health Outcomes of Intensive Mothering." *Journal of Child and Family Studies* 22, no. 5 (2013): 614-620.

Robinson, Fiona. "Discourses of Motherhood and Women's Health: Maternal Thinking as Feminist Politics." *Journal of International Political Theory* 10, no. 1 (2014): 94-108.

Robson, Colin. *Real World Research*. Wiley, 2011.

Root-Bernstein, Robert Scott, and Michele Root-Bernstein. *Sparks of Genius: The Thirteen Thinking Tools of the World's Most Creative People*. Houghton Mifflin Harcourt, 2001.

Ruddick, Sara. *Maternal Thinking: Toward a Politics of Peace*. Beacon Press, 1995.

Sciberras, Danica. *Pregnant Women's Expectations for the Early Postpartum Period after Their First Childbirth*. BS thesis. University of Malta, 2022.

Segrin, Chris, Michelle Givertz, Paulina Swaitkowski, and Neil Montgomery. "Overparenting is Associated with Child Problems and a Critical Family Environment." *Journal of Child and Family Studies* 24, no. 2 (2015): 470-479.

Shaver, Phillip R., Mario Mikulincer, Shiri Lavy, and Jude Cassidy. "Understanding and Altering Hurt Feelings: An Attachment-theoretical Perspective on the Generation and Regulation of Emotions." In *Feeling Hurt in Close Relationships*, edited by Antia L. Vangelisti, 92-119. Cambridge University Press.

Sheehy, Gail. *Passages*. Ballantine Books, 2006.

Shlain, Leonard. *The Alphabet Versus the Goddess: The Conflict between Word and Image*. Penguin, 1999.

Siegel, Daniel. *Parenting From the Inside Out: How a Deeper Self-Understanding Can Help You Raise Children*. Tarcher, 2013.

Small, Meredith. *Our Babies, Ourselves: How Biology and Culture Shape the Way We Parent.* Anchor, 1999.

Smith, Jonathan A. "Towards a Relational Self: Social Engagement during Pregnancy and Psychological Preparation for Motherhood." *British Journal of Social Psychology* 38, no. 4 (1999).

Springgay, Stephanie, and Debra Freedman. *Mothering A Bodied Curriculum.* Univeristy of Toronto Press, 2012.

Starr, Mirabai. *Saint Teresa of Avila: Passionate Mystic.* Sounds True, 2013.

Strand, Clark, and Perdita Finn. *The Way of the Rose: The Radical Path of the Divine Feminine Hidden in the Rosary.* Random House, 2019.

Strand, Sophie. *The Madonna Secret.* Bear and Co., 2023.

Swigart, Jane. *The Myth of the Bad Mother: The Emotional Realities of Mothering.* Doubleday, 1991.

Tavris, Carol. *Anger: The Misunderstood Emotion.* Touchstone, 1989.

Taylor, Jill Bolte. *Whole Brain Living: The Anatomy of Choice and the Four Characters That Drive Our Life.* Hay House, 2021.

Teeffelen, Ans, et al. "Women Want Proactive Psychosocial Support from Midwives During Transition to Motherhood: a Qualitative Study." *Midwifery*, 2009: 1-6.

Thomasson, Melissa A., and Jaret Treber. "From Home to Hospital: The Evolution of Childbirth in the United States, 1928–1940." *Explorations in Economic History* 45, no. 1 (2008): 76-99.

Thurer, Shari L. *The Myths of Motherhood: How Culture Reinvents the Good Mother*. Penguin Books, 1994.

Trad, Paul V. "On Becoming a Mother: In the Throes of Developmental Transformation" *Psychoanalytic Psychology* 7, no. 3 (1990): 341-361.

Tsabary, Shefali. *The Conscious Parent: Transforming Ourselves, Empowering Our Children*. Hachette UK, 2014.

Walks, Michelle, and Naomi McPherson. *An Anthropology of Mothering*. Demeter Press, 2011.

Williams, J. Whitridge. "Medical Education and the Midwife Problem in the United States." *Journal of the American Medical Association* 58, no. 1 (1912): 1-7.

Williamson, Marianne. *A Woman's Worth*. Ballantine Books, 1994.

Winter, Gayan Silvie, and Jo Dose. *Vision Quest Tarot*. AGM-Urania; Cards edition, 1999.

Zaidi, Zeenat F. "Gender Differences in Human Brain: A Review." *The Open Anatomy Journal* 2, no. 1 (2010).

About Dr. Gertrude Lyons

Dr. Gertrude Lyons has dedicated her career to unlocking the natural ability of individuals to expand and awaken to their power. Her advocacy for rethinking motherhood as a creative force that influences every part of an individual's life is informed by her Doctorate and two master's degrees, where she authentically explored her own mothering journey.

Dr. Lyons launched her podcast, *Rewrite the Mother Code*, in 2020 to facilitate candid conversations while offering practical tools that inspire listeners to explore what it means to mother— not only children but also their potential, relationships, and goals.

With over 25 years of experience helping individuals, couples, and families, Dr. Lyons, partnering with her husband, opened a retreat center in Mexico. She creates supportive and dynamic spaces for participants to honor destruction and creation, shedding and releasing what no longer serves them while embracing their innate wisdom and new possibilities. Her work has been featured in books, articles, lectures, podcasts, radio, and TV appearances.

Gertrude's journey has been shaped by profound personal awakenings in sacred spaces worldwide, from Nepal's Himalayan temples to the healing waters of Laos. Whether focusing one-on-one through coaching and customized immersive experiences or hosting groups at one of her retreat centers, Dr. Lyons looks to curate opportunities to reflect, reconnect, and take meaningful steps toward living with greater clarity and purpose.

Beyond her professional life, she renews herself by traveling with her husband and family and embracing the joys and challenges of life with curiosity and intention.